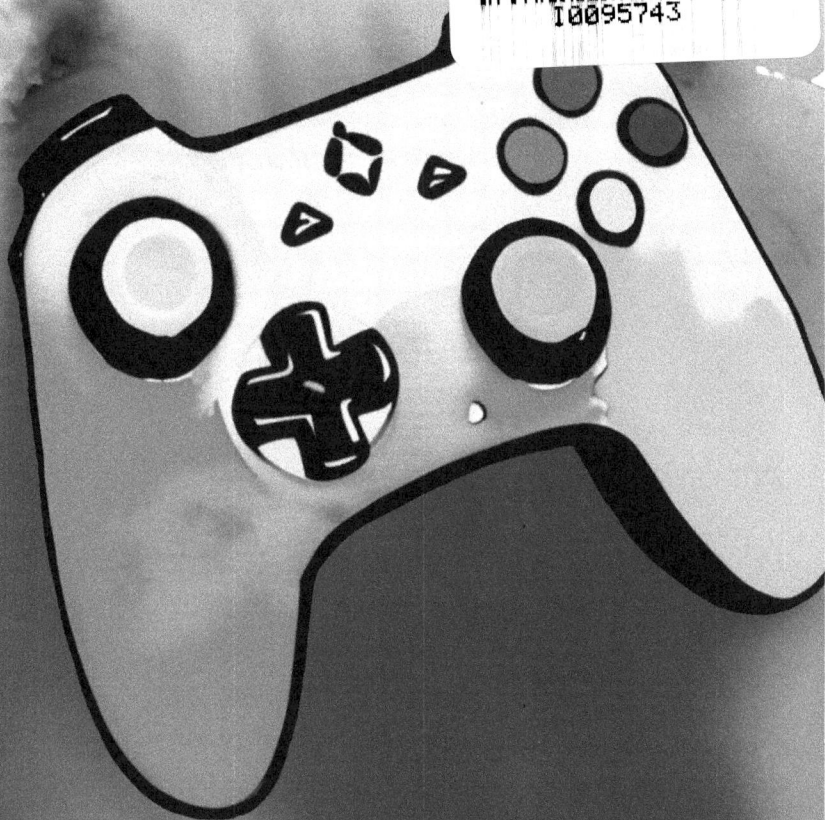

DAILY GRATITUDE
ENCOURAGING AFFIRMATIONS
&
POSITIVE COPING SKILLS

I0095743

I dedicate this workbook to Dylan.
Thank you for sharing your creative ideas with me.

xoxo

Mama Maya

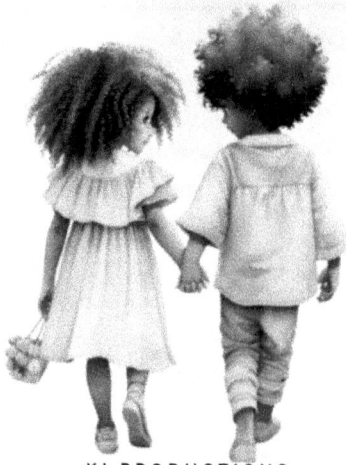

KI PRODUCTIONS
Where every story matters

ISBN: 978-1-961605-46-6
The Neurodivergent Collection

Written, Designed, & Edited by Marya Patrice Sherron

WHAT IS GRATITUDE?

GRATITUDE IS WHEN YOU FEEL THANKFUL FOR THE GOOD THINGS IN YOUR LIFE.

WHAT ARE AFFIRMATIONS?

POSITIVE AFFIRMATIONS ARE IDEAS AND PHRASES THAT HELP US OVERCOME NEGATIVE THOUGHTS AND FEELINGS.

WHAT ARE COPING SKILLS?

COPING SKILLS ARE POSITIVE, HEALTHY WAYS TO RESPOND TO OVERWHELMING AND DIFFICULT EMOTIONS.

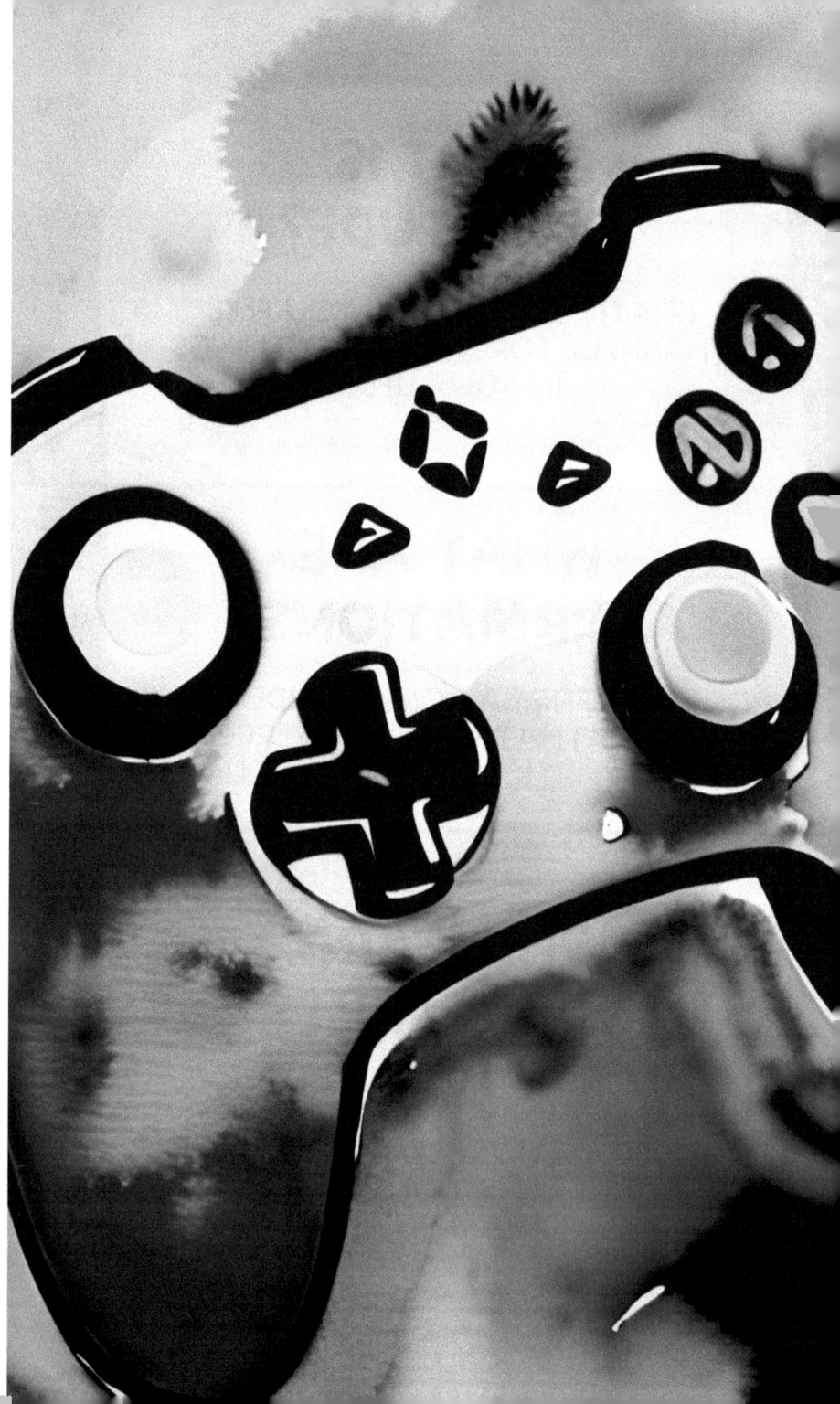

ALL ABOUT ME

My name is _____

I am from _____

I live in _____

This is a picture of me!

My favorite color is

My favorite food is

My favorite tv show is

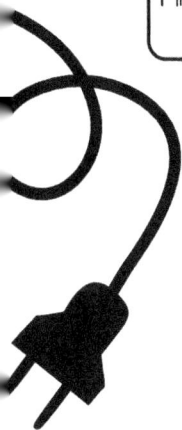

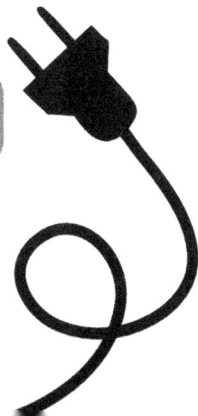

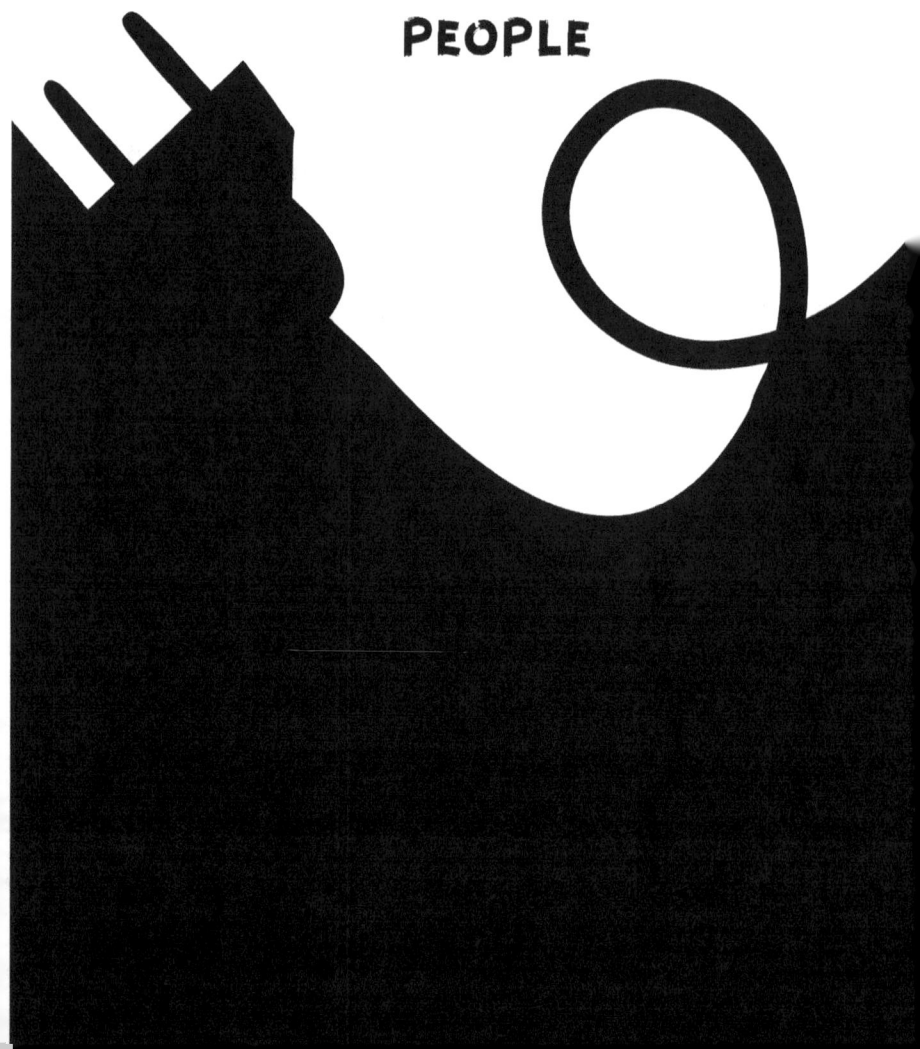

I LIKE ME

&

SO DO OTHER

PEOPLE

DAILY GRATITUDE

What are three things you are grateful for today?

What was the best part of your day?

Who made a difference in your life today?

Describe your overall mood today in 1-3 words.

Today's Date

_____

_____

_____

_____

_____

_____

_____

_____

_____

_____

_____

_____

_____

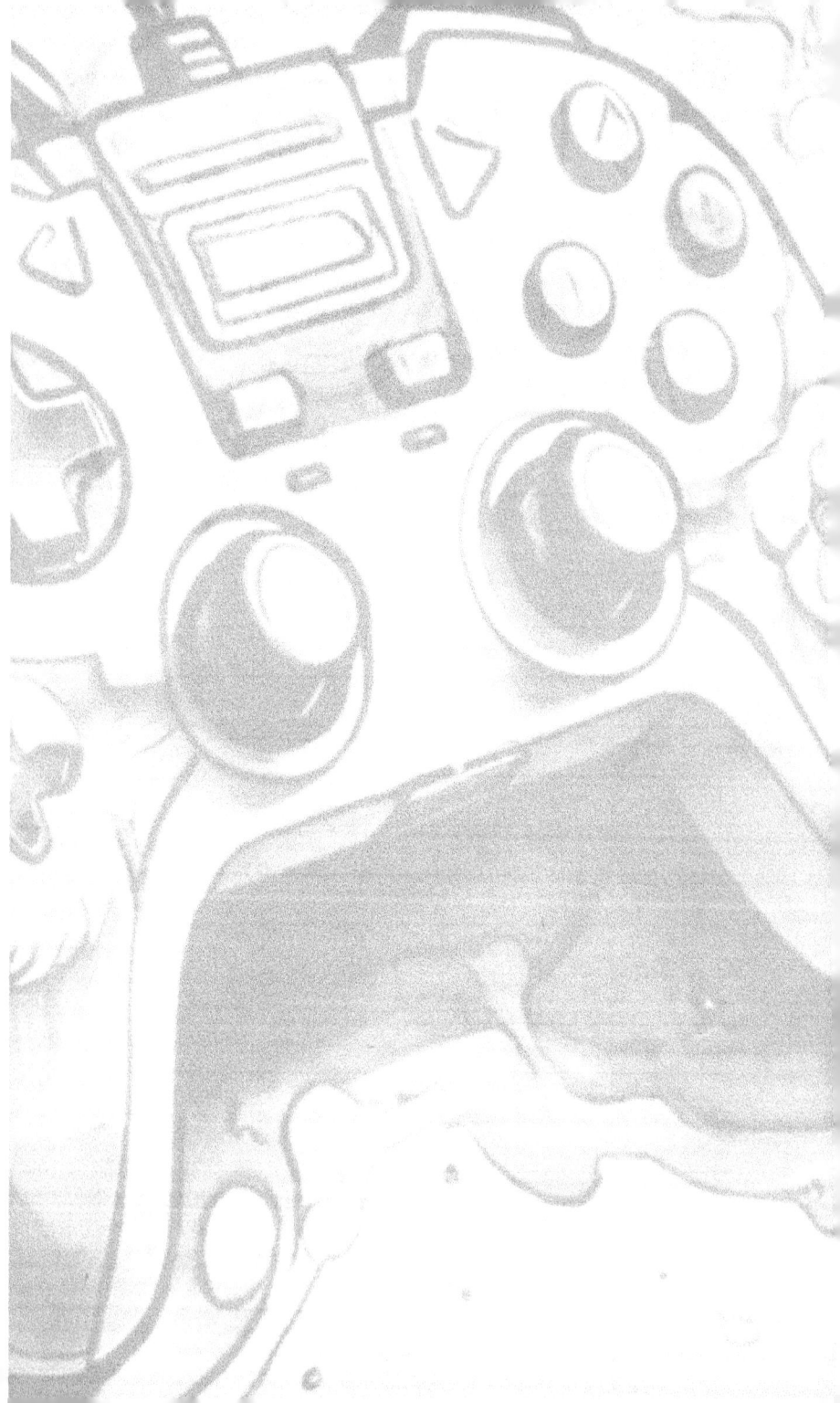

DO A SURVEY

Ask 6 people what they are most grateful for and write their answers below.

MY PROBLEM

HAS A SOLUTION

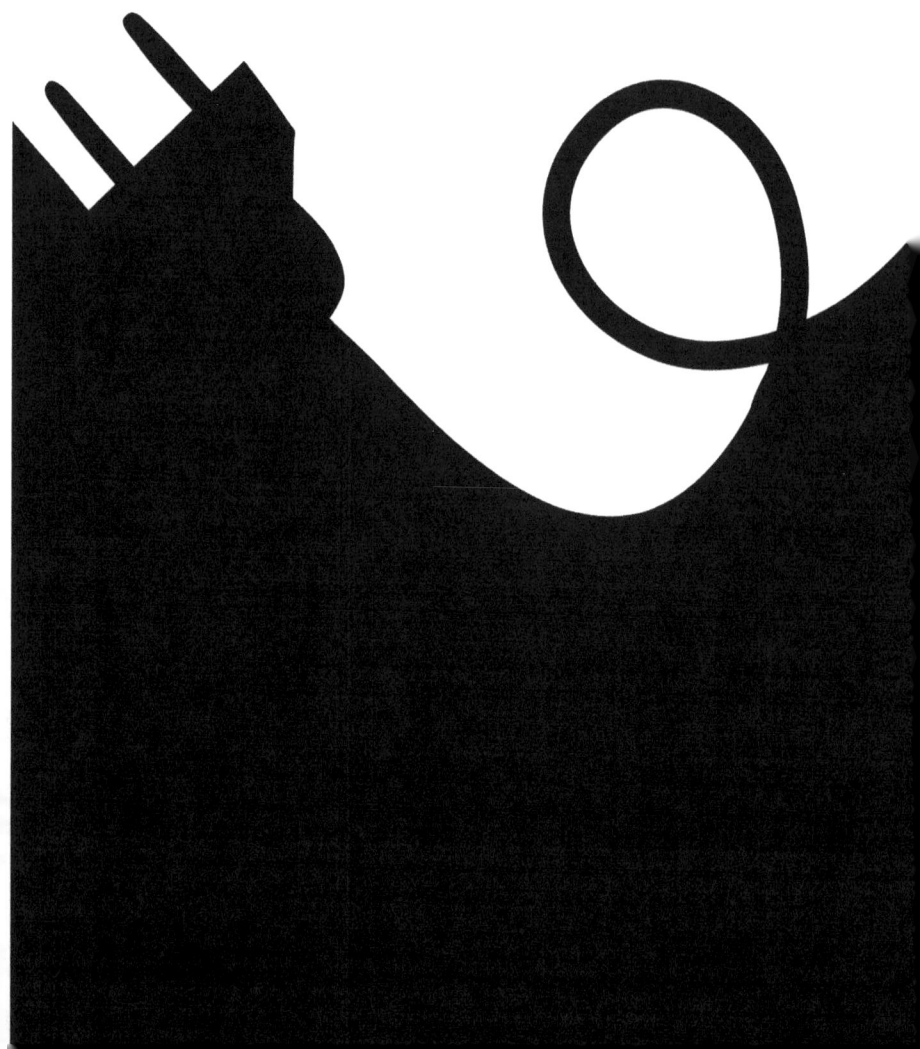

DAILY GRATITUDE

What are three things you are grateful for today?

Who made a difference in your life today?

What was the best part of your day?

Describe your overall mood today in 1-3 words.

Today's Date

DATE

_____

_____

_____

_____

_____

_____

_____

_____

_____

_____

_____

_____

_____

_____

_____

_____

_____

_____

_____

_____

_____

_____

_____

_____

_____

_____

_____

_____

_____

_____

_____

_____

_____

_____

_____

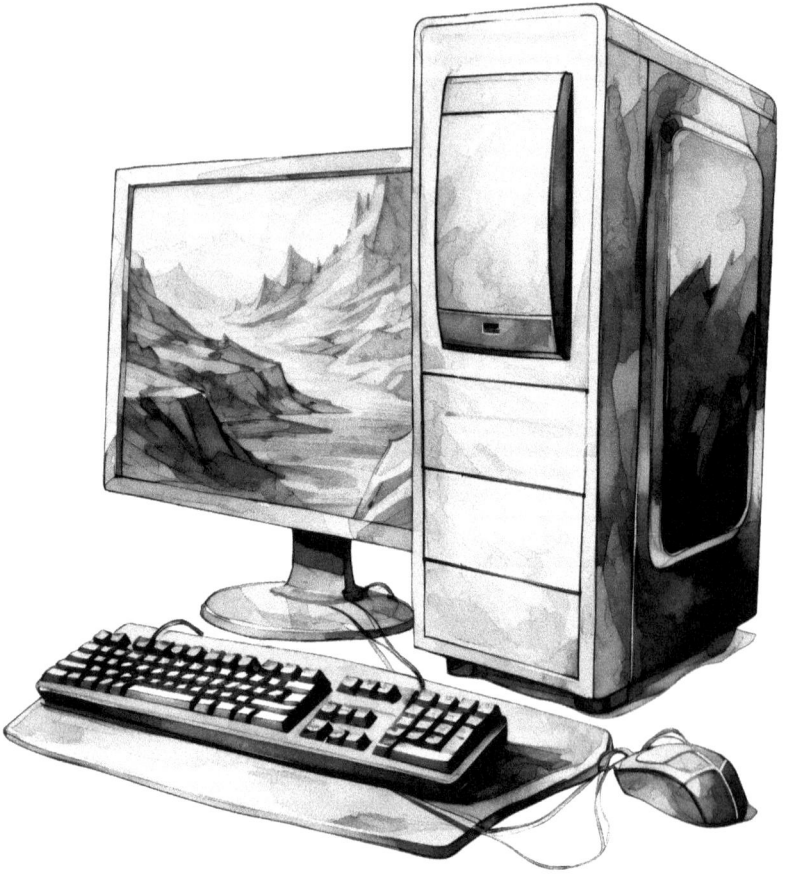

MORE ABOUT ME...

Write a feeling next to each facial expression and then list a few things that make you feel this way.

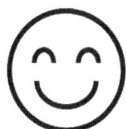 ————————

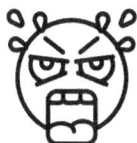 ————————

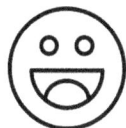 ————————

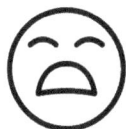 ————————

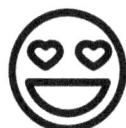 ————————

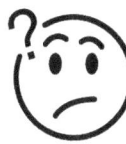 ————————

IT'S OKAY TO ASK FOR HELP

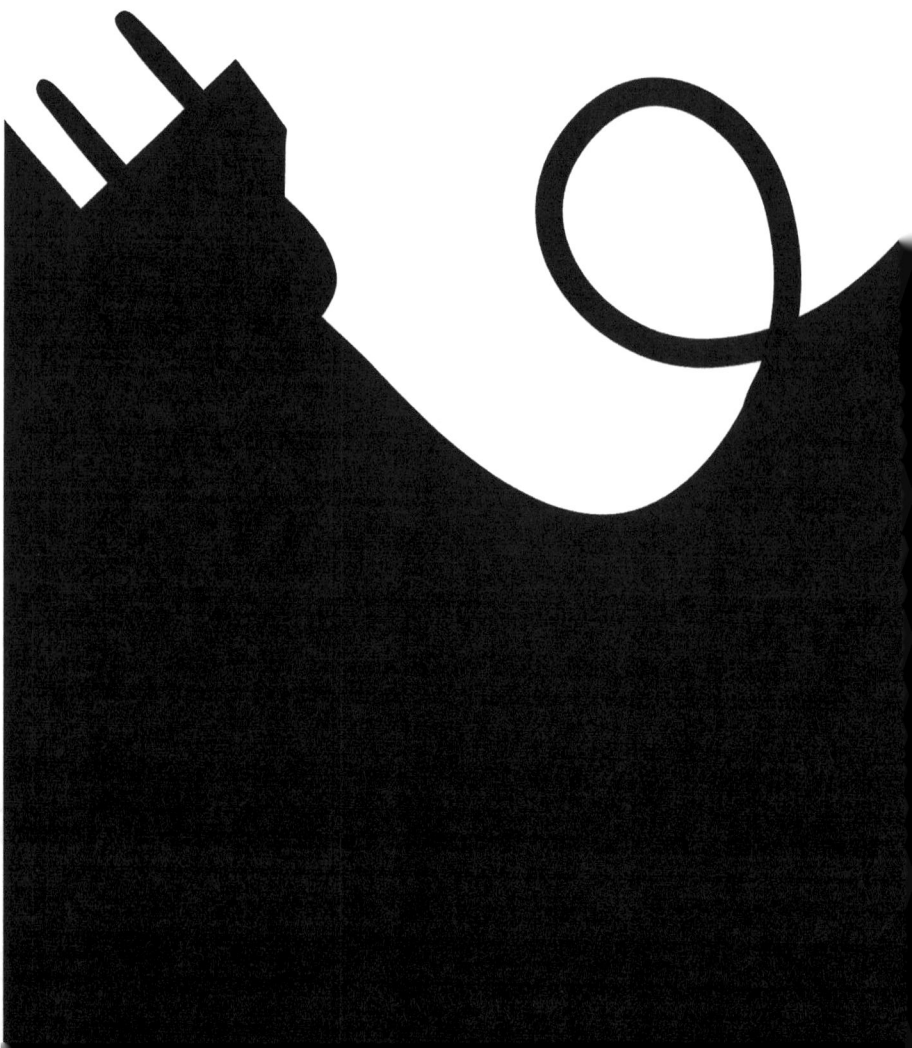

DAILY GRATITUDE

What are three things you are grateful for today?

Who made a difference in your life today?

What was the best part of your day?

Describe your overall mood today in 1-3 words.

Today's Date

I'M STILL GROWING & LEARNING

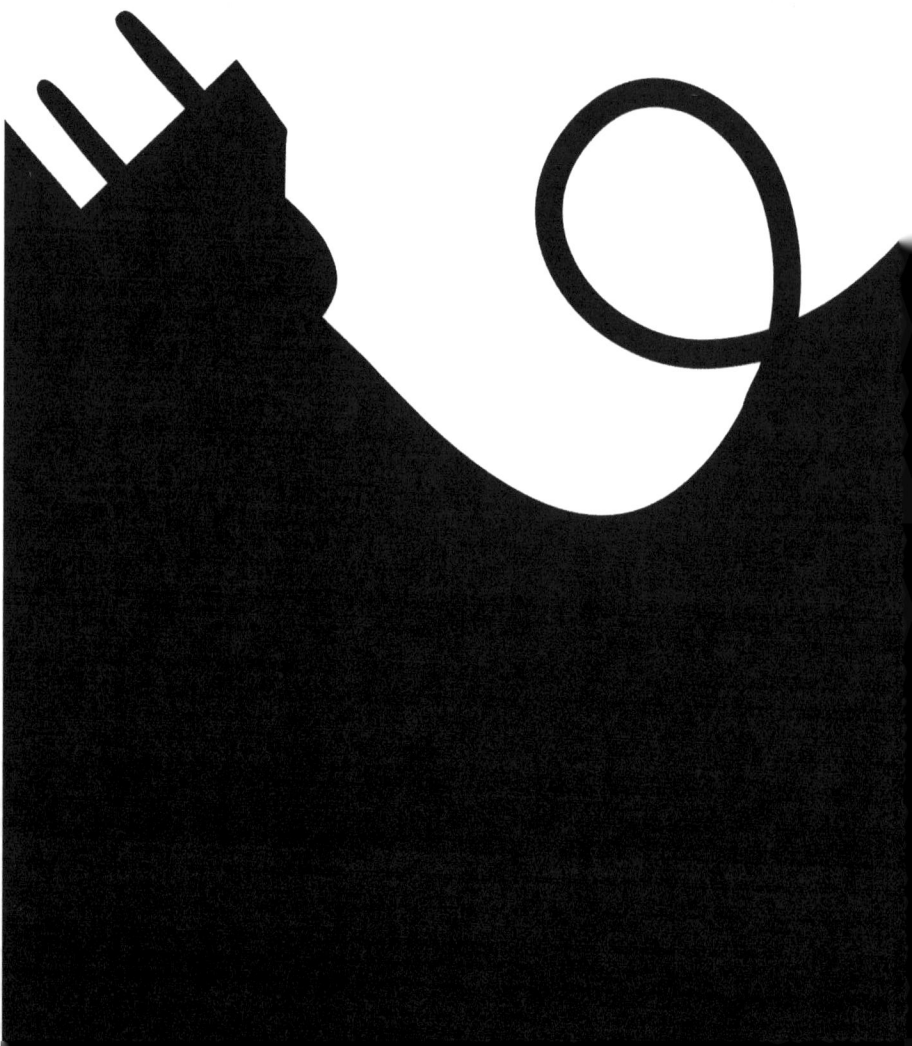

DAILY GRATITUDE

What are three things you are grateful for today?

Who made a difference in your life today?

What was the best part of your day?

Describe your overall mood today in 1-3 words.

Today's Date

SOME DAYS ARE HARDER
THAN OTHERS...
TOMORROW IS A NEW DAY.

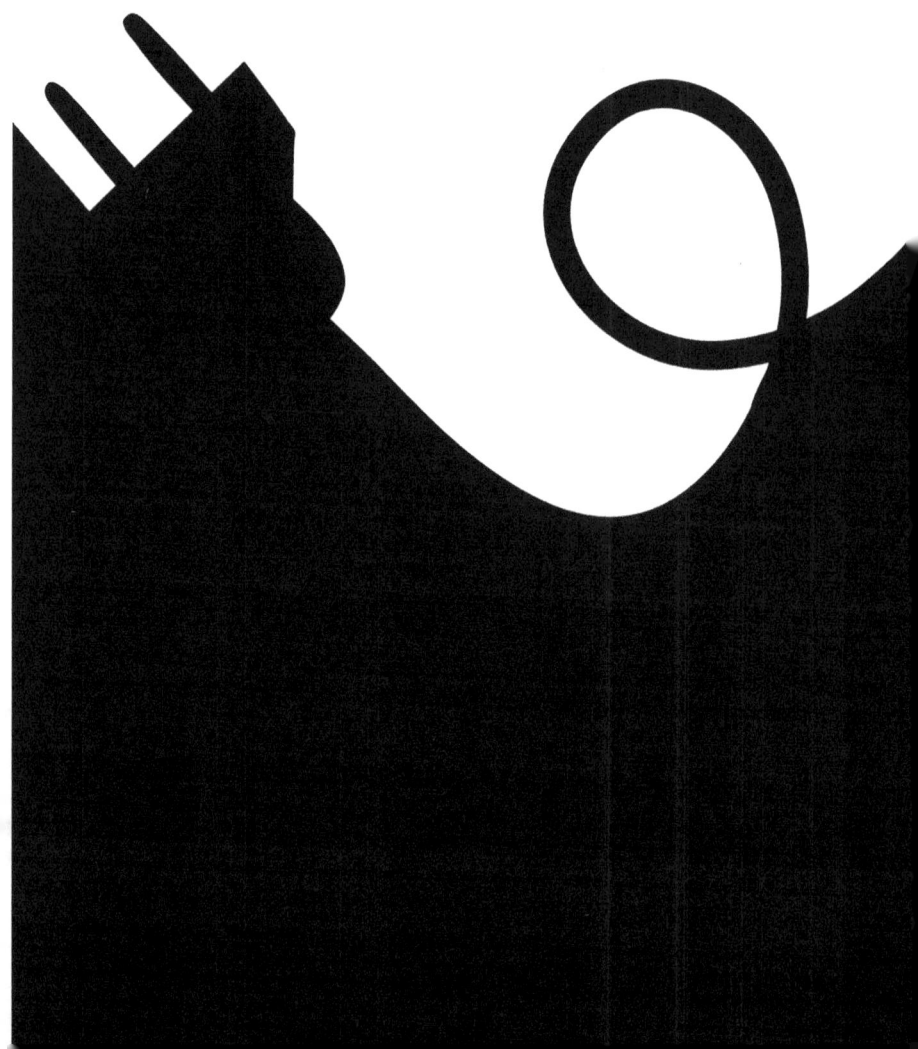

DAILY GRATITUDE

What are three things you are grateful for today?

Who made a difference in your life today?

What was the best part of your day?

Describe your overall mood today in 1-3 words.

Today's Date

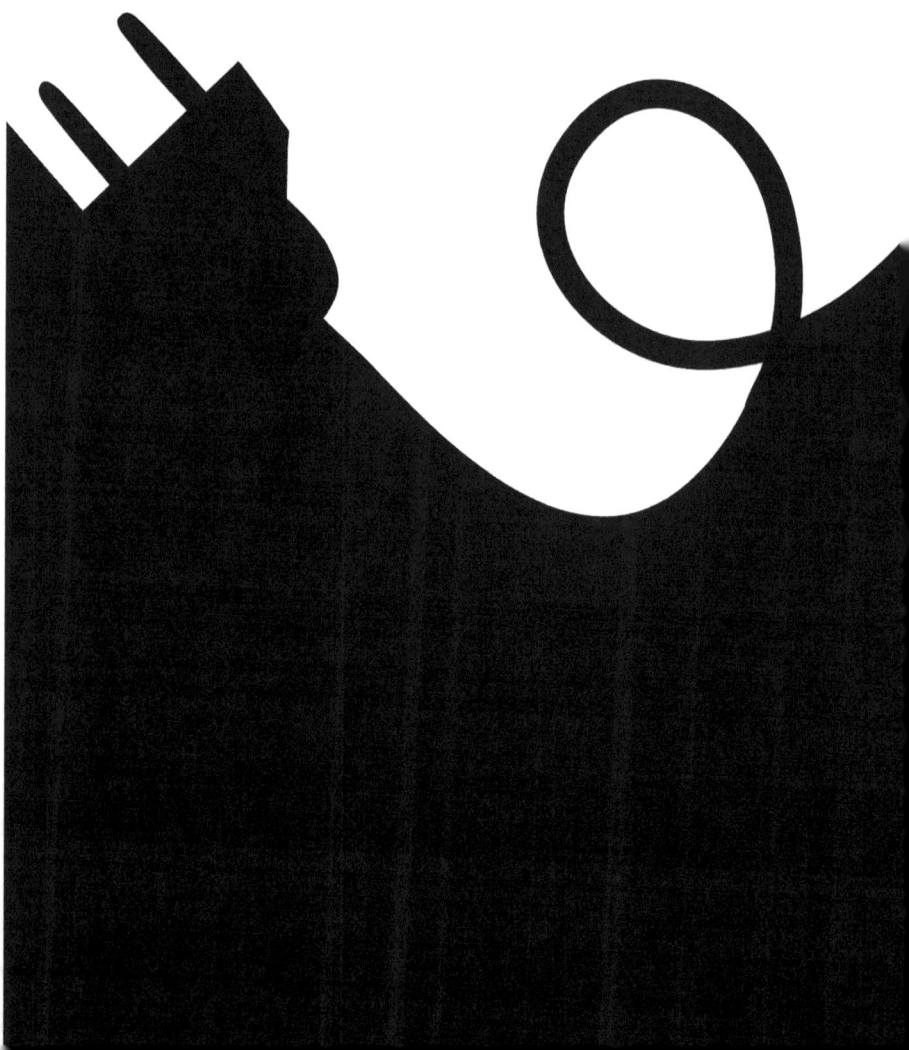

I CAN DO HARD

THINGS

DAILY GRATITUDE

What are three things you are grateful for today?

Who made a difference in your life today?

What was the best part of your day?

Describe your overall mood today in 1-3 words.

Today's Date

_____

_____

_____

_____

_____

_____

_____

_____

_____

_____

_____

_____

_____

_____

_____

_____

_____

_____

_____

My family believes in me

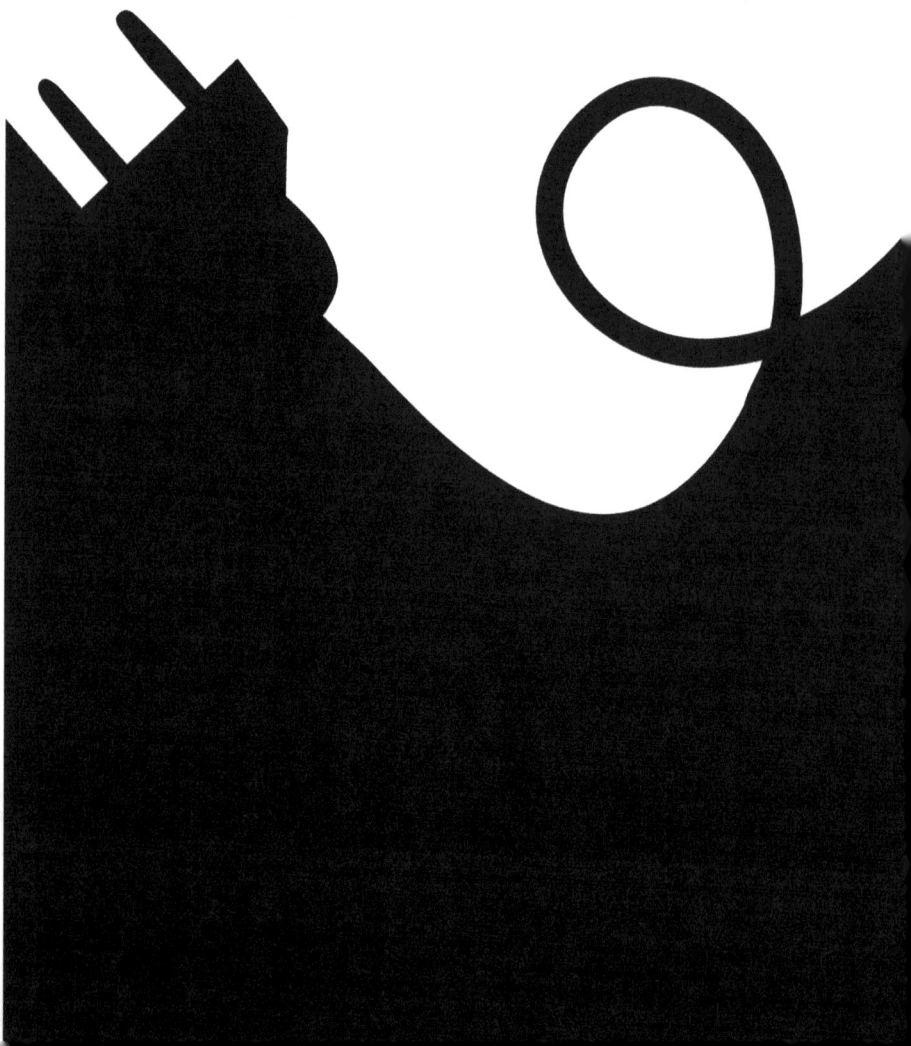

DAILY GRATITUDE

What are three things you are grateful for today?

Who made a difference in your life today?

What was the best part of your day?

Describe your overall mood today in 1-3 words.

Today's Date

_____

_____

_____

_____

_____

_____

_____

_____

_____

_____

_____

_____

_____

_____

_____

_____

_____

_____

_____

_____

_____

_____

_____

_____

_____

_____

_____

_____

_____

_____

_____

_____

_____

_____

I BELIEVE IN

MYSELF

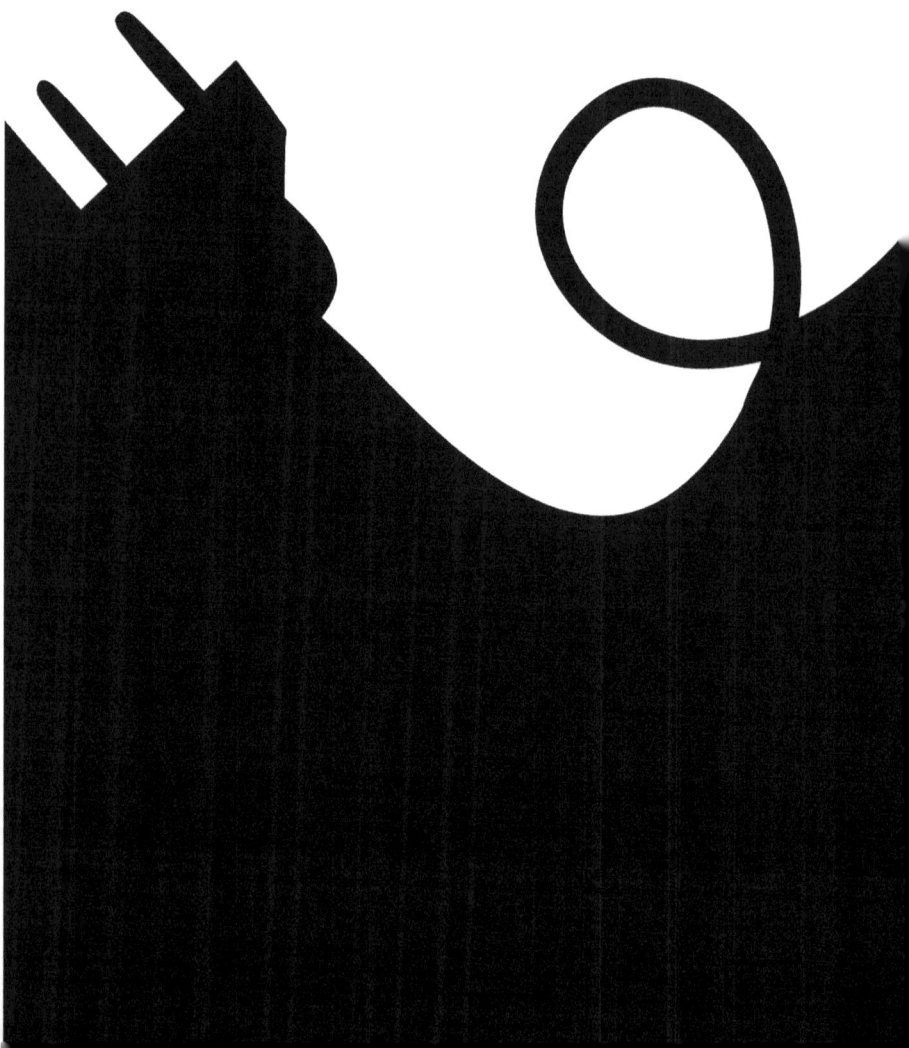

DAILY GRATITUDE

What are three things you are grateful for today?

Who made a difference in your life today?

What was the best part of your day?

Describe your overall mood today in 1-3 words.

Today's Date

WHAT MAKES YOU FEEL ANXIETY?

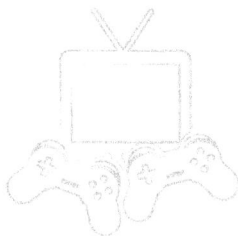

THINGS I CAN DO WHEN I FEEL ANXIOUS

- ☐ think of 3 positive thoughts
- ☐ go for a walk
- ☐ talk with someone you trust
- ☐ write down how you are feeling
- ☐ listen to calming music
- ☐ ....
- ☐ ....
- ☐ ....
- ☐ ....
- ☐ ....

ADD A FEW THINGS OF YOUR OWN THAT HELP YOU RELAX & STAY CALM.

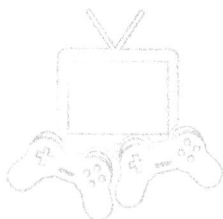

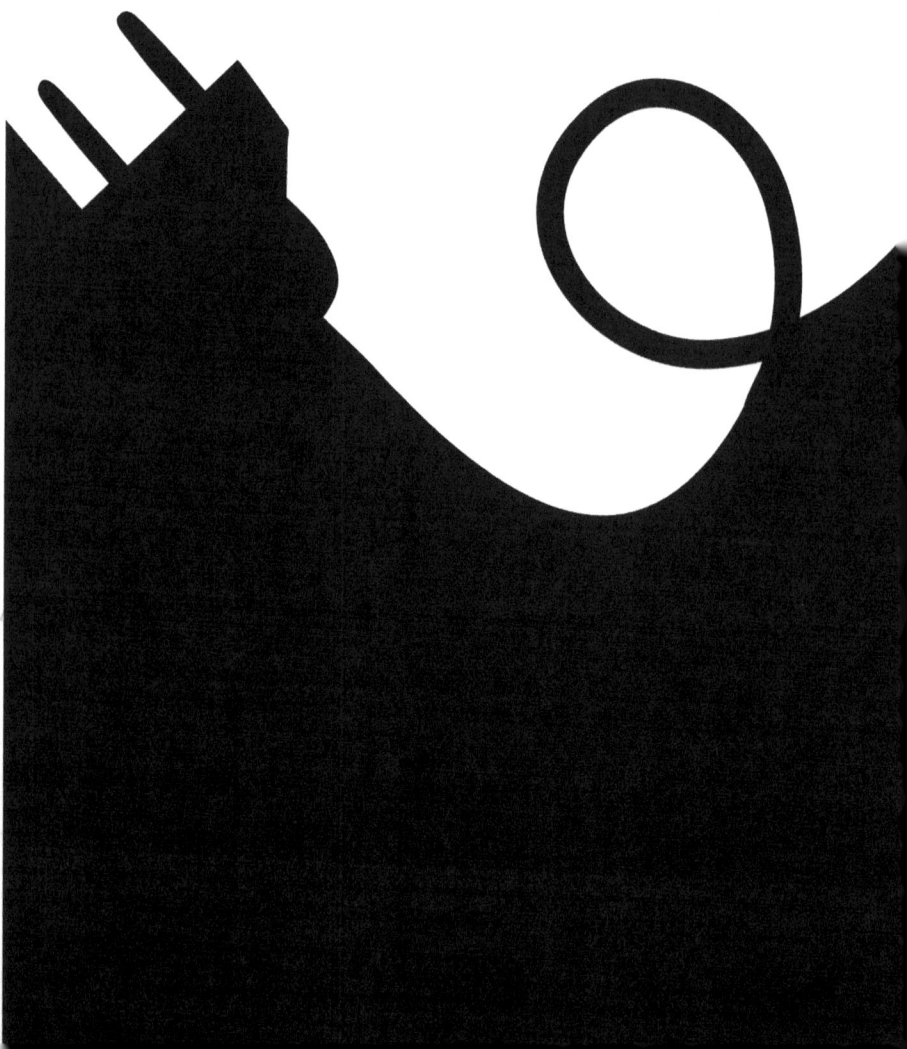

I CAN LEARN

NEW THINGS

DAILY GRATITUDE

What are three things you are grateful for today?

Who made a difference in your life today?

What was the best part of your day?

Describe your overall mood today in 1-3 words.

Today's Date

_____

_____

_____

_____

_____

_____

_____

_____

_____

_____

_____

_____

_____

_____

_____

_____

_____

_____

_____

_____

_____

_____

_____

_____

_____

_____

_____

_____

_____

_____

_____

_____

I CAN HELP
OTHERS HAVE A
GREAT DAY

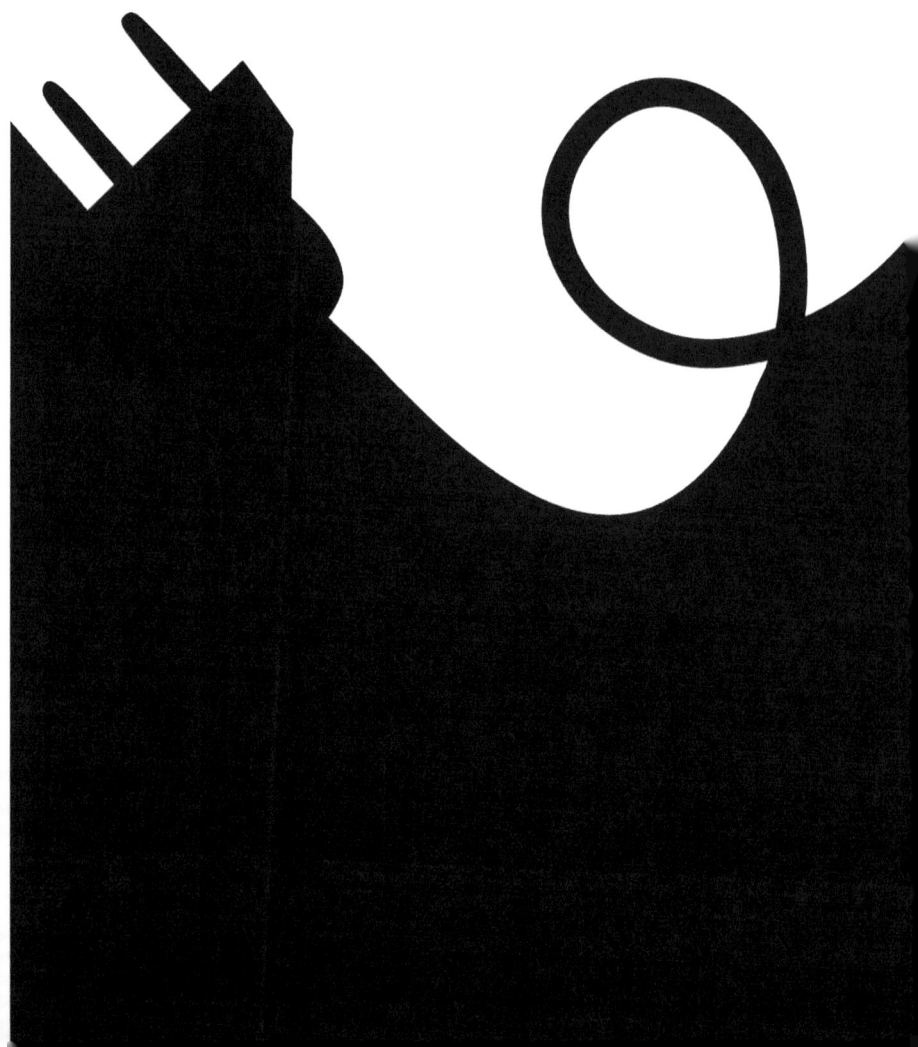

DAILY GRATITUDE

What are three things you are grateful for today?

Who made a difference in your life today?

What was the best part of your day?

Describe your overall mood today in 1-3 words.

Today's Date

_____

_____

_____

_____

_____

_____

_____

_____

_____

_____

_____

_____

_____

I GET TO
CHOOSE MY
MOOD TODAY

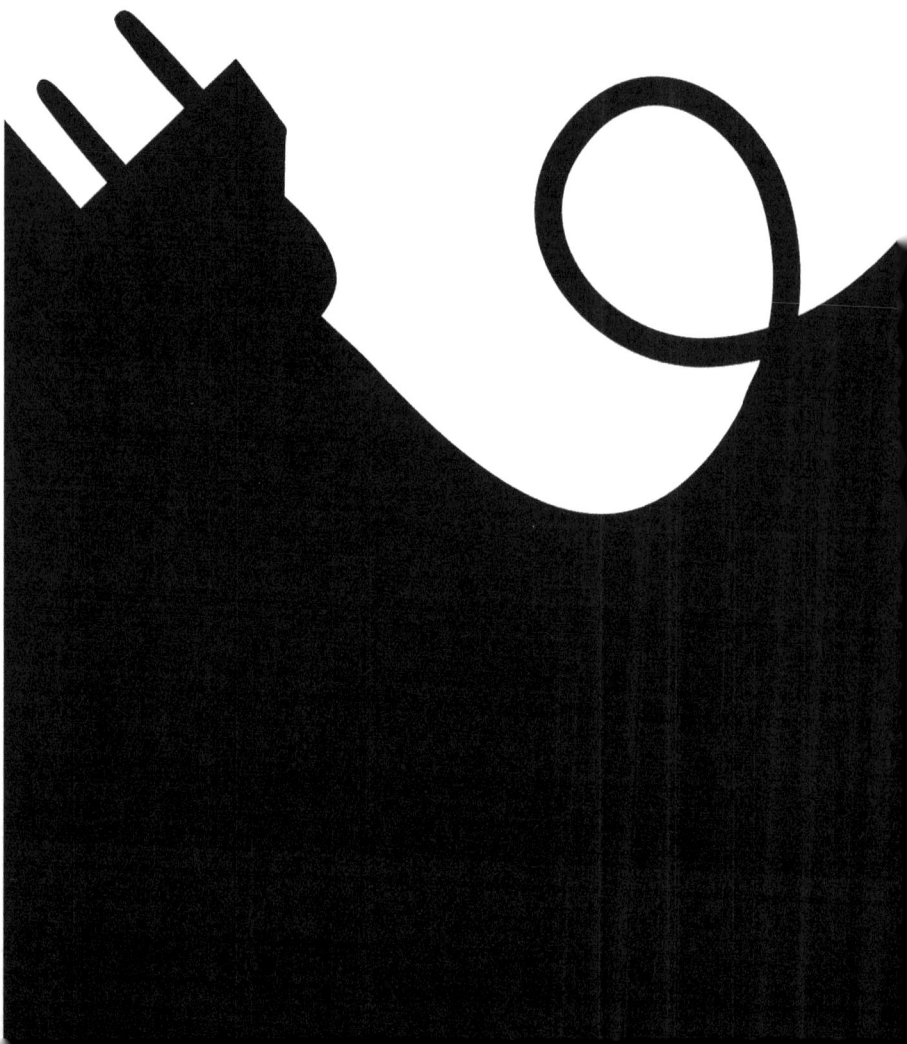

BEING GRATEFUL FOR FAMILY

Name one person you are grateful for.

Draw or tape a picture of them below.

Write three things you like about this person.

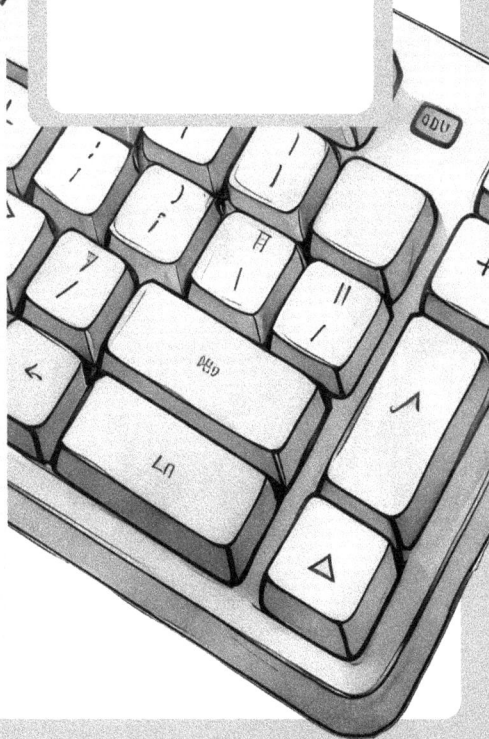

_____

_____

_____

_____

_____

_____

_____

_____

_____

_____

_____

_____

I.AM.COURAGEOUS

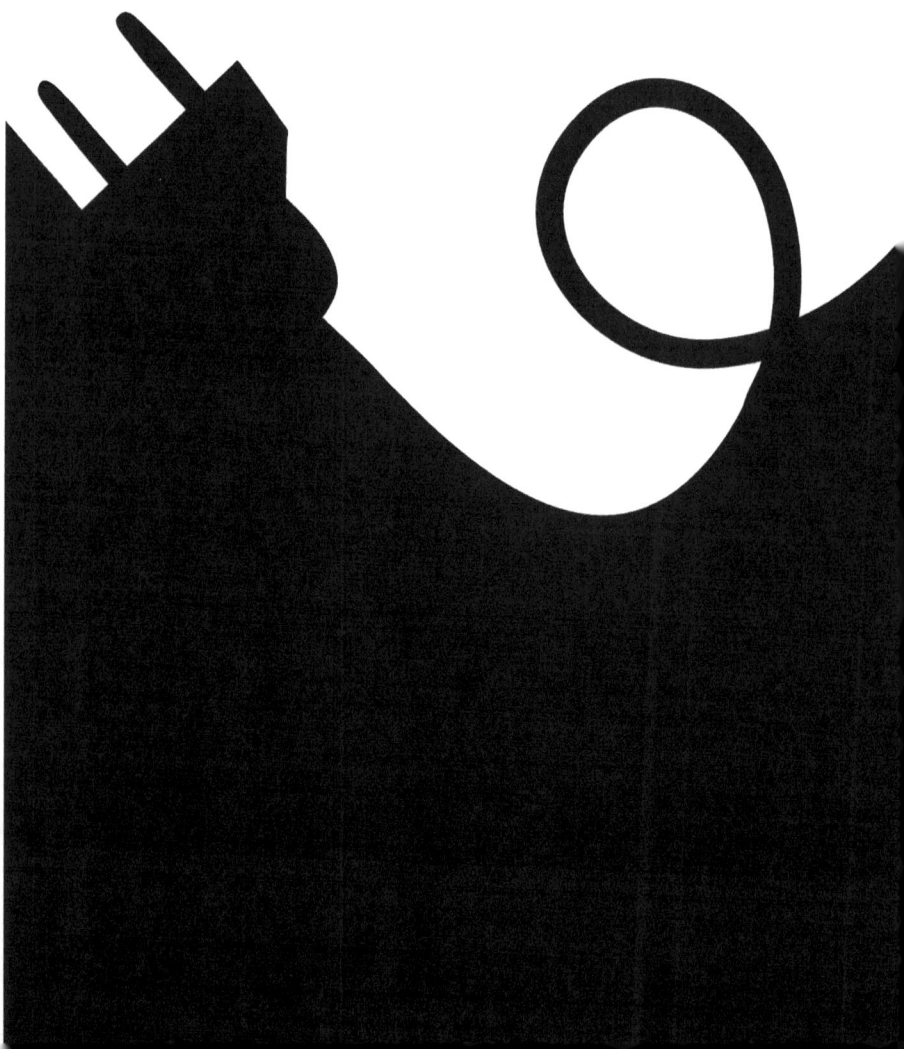

DAILY GRATITUDE

What are three things you are grateful for today?

Who made a difference in your life today?

What was the best part of your day?

Describe your overall mood today in 1-3 words.

Today's Date

_____

_____

_____

_____

_____

_____

_____

_____

_____

_____

_____

_____

_____

_____

_____

_____

_____

_____

_____

_____

_____

_____

_____

_____

_____

_____

_____

_____

_____

_____

_____

TODAY, ASK SOMEONE TO SHARE THEIR FAVORITE
AFFIRMATION & WRITE IT ABOVE.

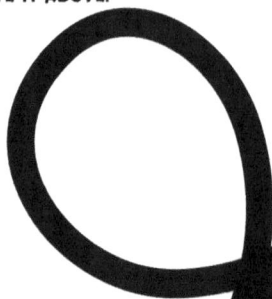

DAILY GRATITUDE

What are three things you are grateful for today?

Who made a difference in your life today?

What was the best part of your day?

Describe your overall mood today in 1-3 words.

Today's Date

_____

_____

_____

_____

_____

_____

_____

_____

_____

_____

_____

_____

_____

IT'S OKAY TO
TAKE A BREAK

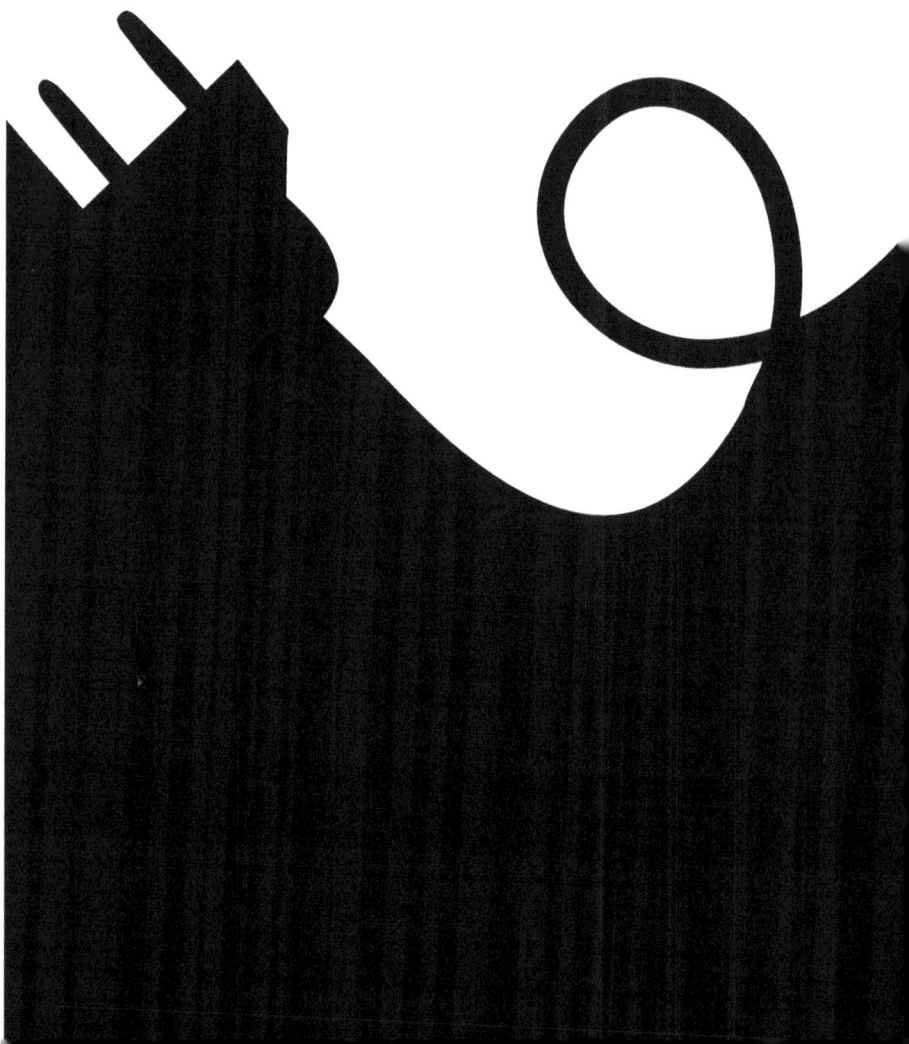

DAILY GRATITUDE

What are three things you are grateful for today?

Who made a difference in your life today?

What was the best part of your day?

Describe your overall mood today in 1-3 words.

Today's Date

_____

_____

_____

_____

_____

_____

_____

_____

_____

_____

_____

_____

_____

_____

_____

_____

_____

_____

_____

_____

_____

_____

_____

_____

_____

_____

_____

_____

_____

_____

_____

_____

TODAY, WRITE YOUR OWN AFFIRMATION IN
THE SPACE ABOVE.

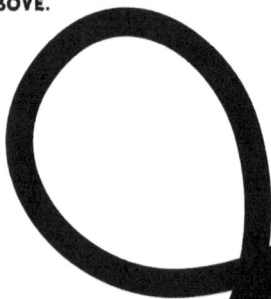

DAILY GRATITUDE

What are three things you are grateful for today?

Who made a difference in your life today?

What was the best part of your day?

Describe your overall mood today in 1-3 words.

Today's Date

_____

_____

_____

_____

_____

_____

_____

_____

_____

_____

_____

_____

_____

_____

_____

TODAY I WILL FOCUS ON ALL THE PEOPLE WHO CARE FOR ME

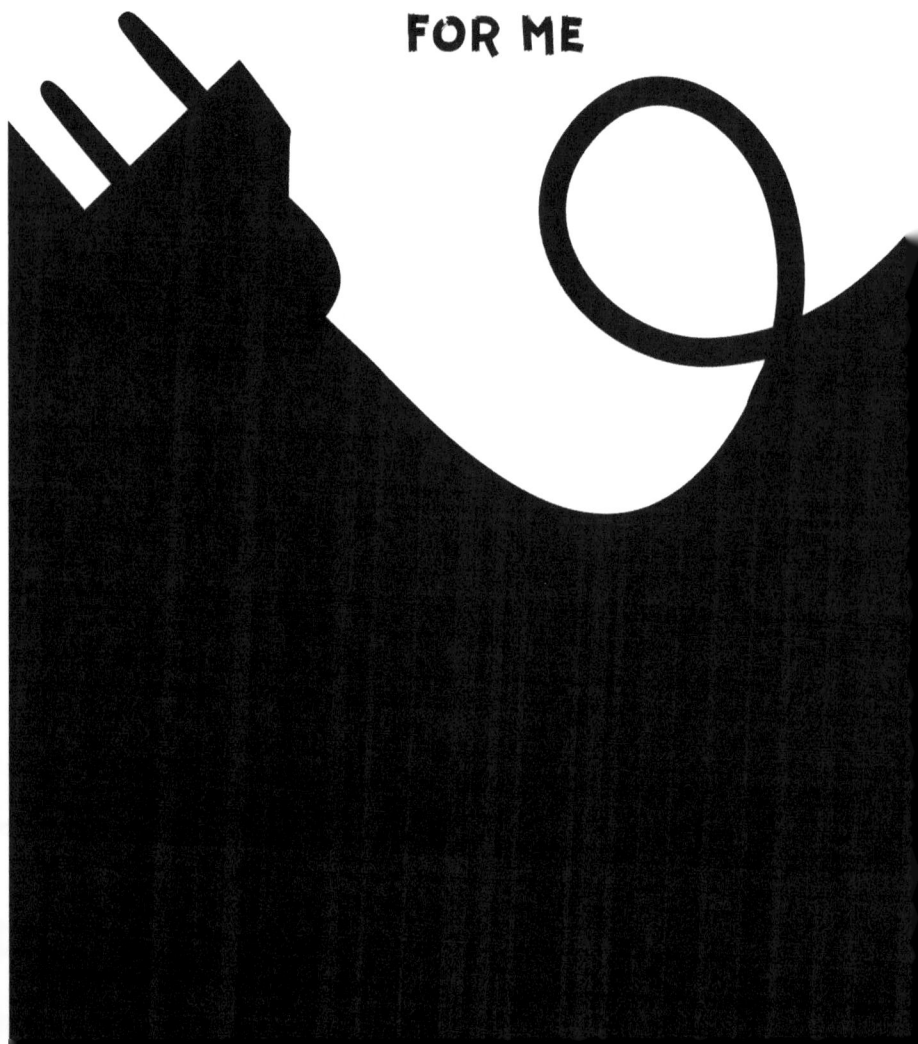

DAILY GRATITUDE

What are three things you are grateful for today?

Who made a difference in your life today?

What was the best part of your day?

Describe your overall mood today in 1-3 words.

Today's Date

_____

_____

_____

_____

_____

_____

_____

_____

_____

_____

_____

_____

_____

_____

TODAY I WILL
TRY SOMETHING
NEW

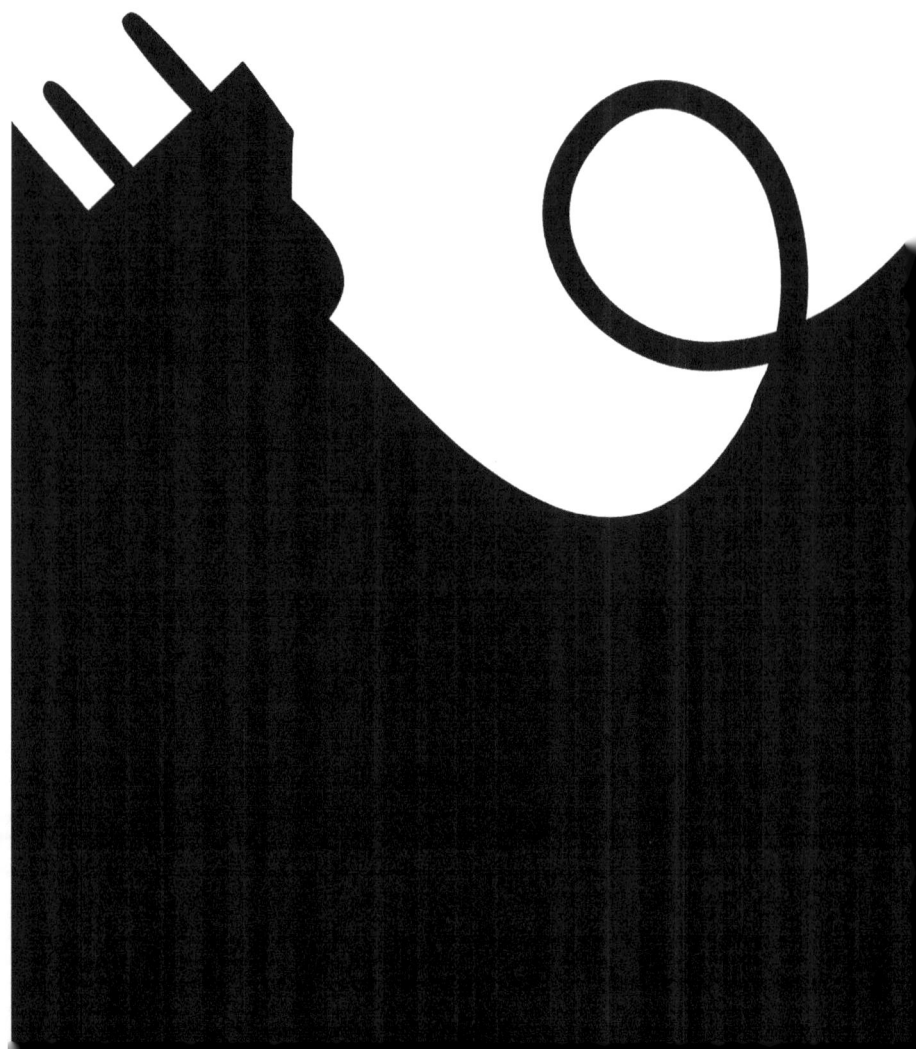

DAILY GRATITUDE

What are three things you are grateful for today?

Who made a difference in your life today?

What was the best part of your day?

Describe your overall mood today in 1-3 words.

Today's Date

_____

_____

_____

_____

_____

_____

_____

_____

_____

_____

_____

_____

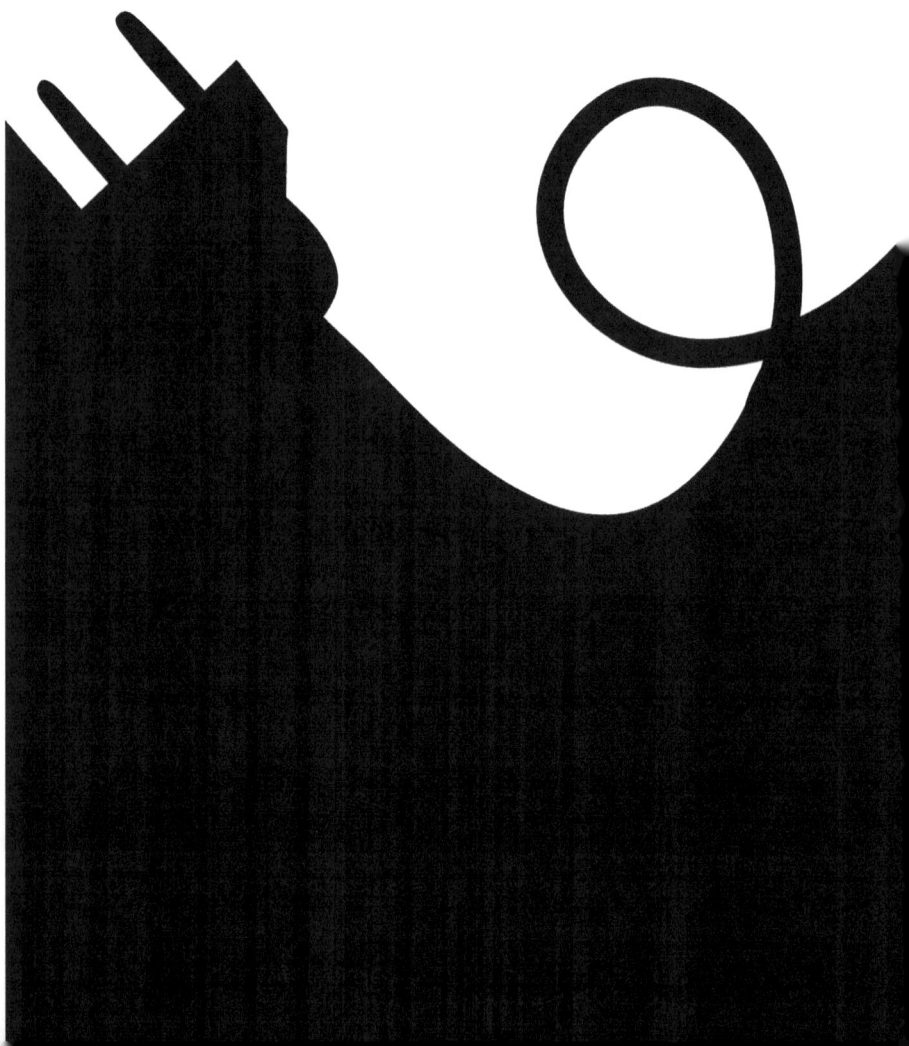

TODAY I CHOOSE

HAPPY THOUGHTS

DAILY GRATITUDE

What are three things you are grateful for today?

Who made a difference in your life today?

What was the best part of your day?

Describe your overall mood today in 1-3 words.

Today's Date

_____

_____

_____

_____

_____

_____

_____

_____

_____

_____

_____

_____

_____

I GET FRUSTRATED WHEN...

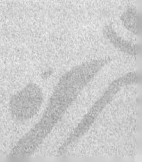

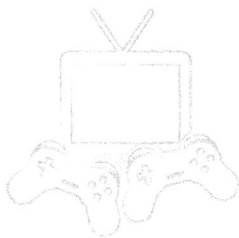

THINGS I CAN
DO WHEN I AM
FRUSTRATED

- ☐ find a new activity to work on
- ☐ smile
- ☐ tell someone that I am frustrated
- ☐ tell someone if I need a break
- ☐ splash cold water on my face
- ☐ ....
- ☐ ....
- ☐ ....
- ☐ ....
- ☐ ....

ADD A FEW
THINGS OF YOUR
OWN THAT CAN
HELP YOU WHEN
YOU'RE FEELING
FRUSTRATED

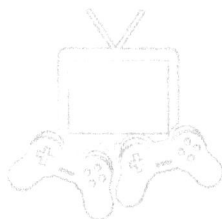

IT'S OKAY TO ASK FOR MORE TIME

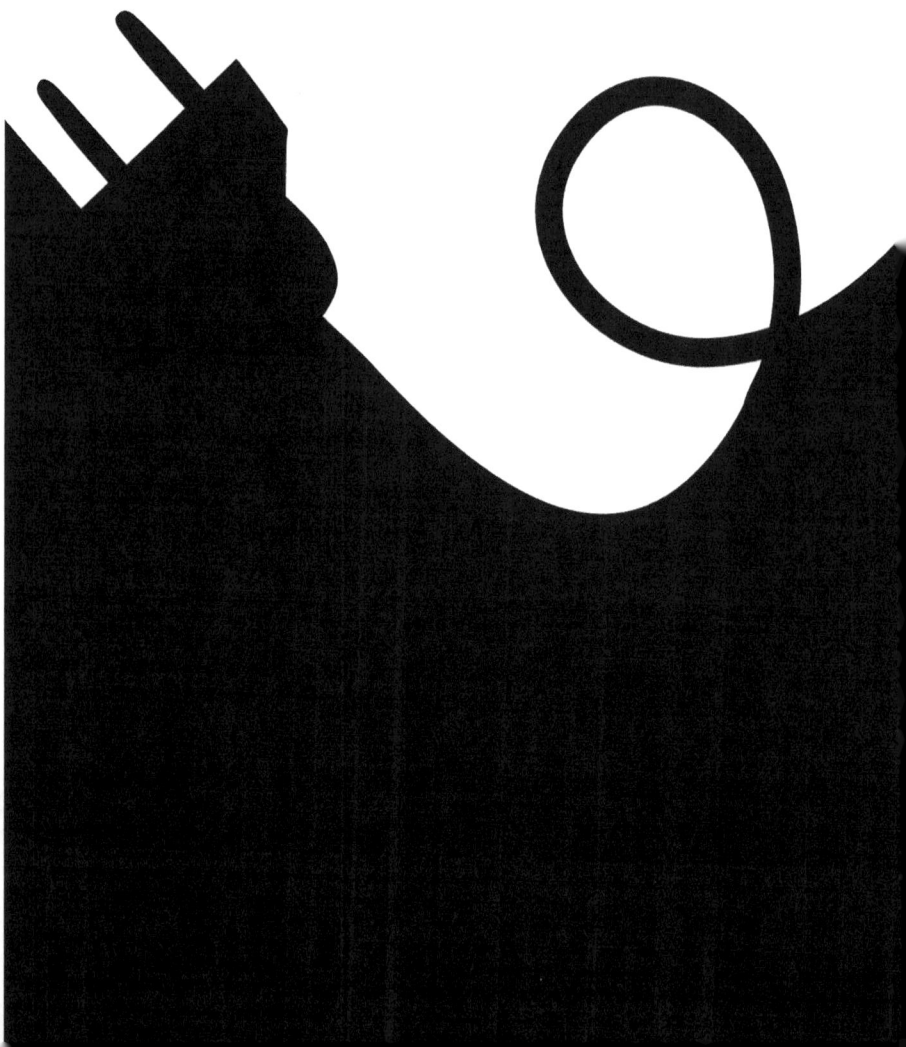

DAILY GRATITUDE

What are three things you are grateful for today?

Who made a difference in your life today?

What was the best part of your day?

Describe your overall mood today in 1-3 words.

Today's Date

_____

_____

_____

_____

_____

_____

_____

_____

_____

_____

_____

_____

I WILL CELEBRATE
THE WAYS I AM
DIFFERENT

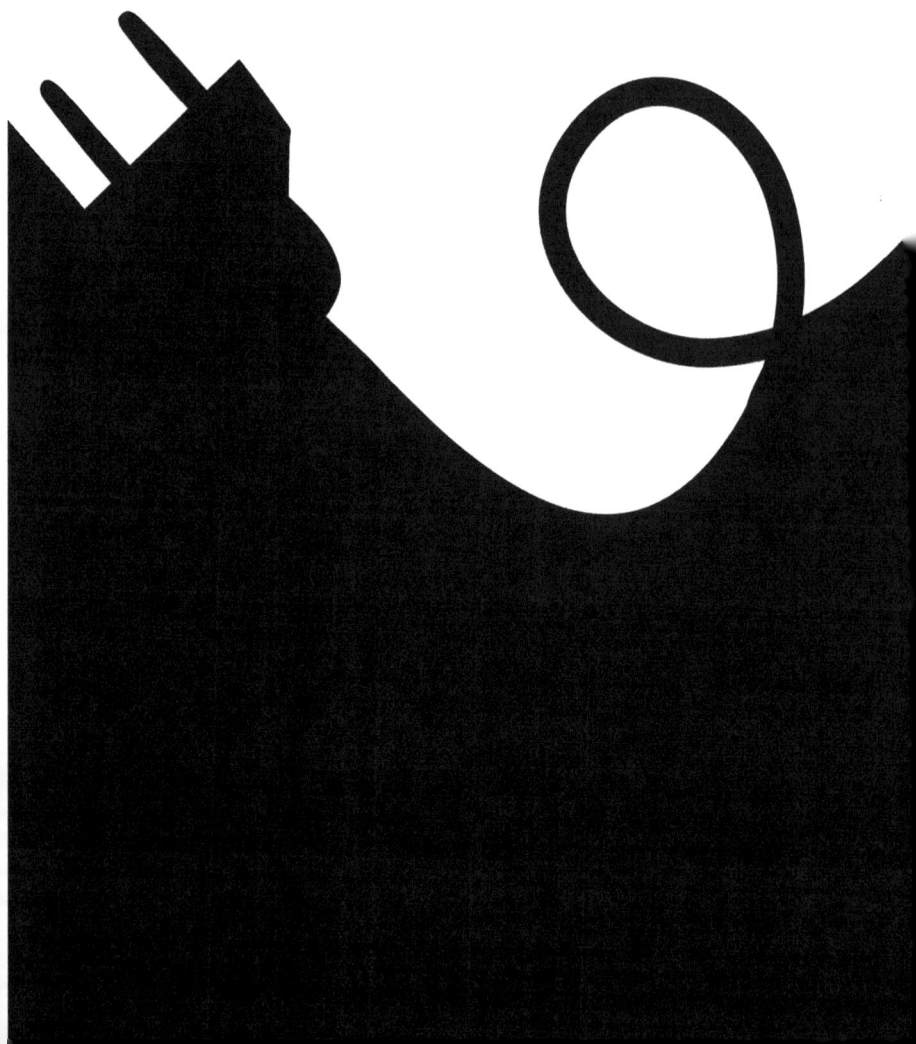

DAILY GRATITUDE

What are three things you are grateful for today?

Who made a difference in your life today?

What was the best part of your day?

Describe your overall mood today in 1-3 words.

Today's Date

I CAN REACH MY GOALS

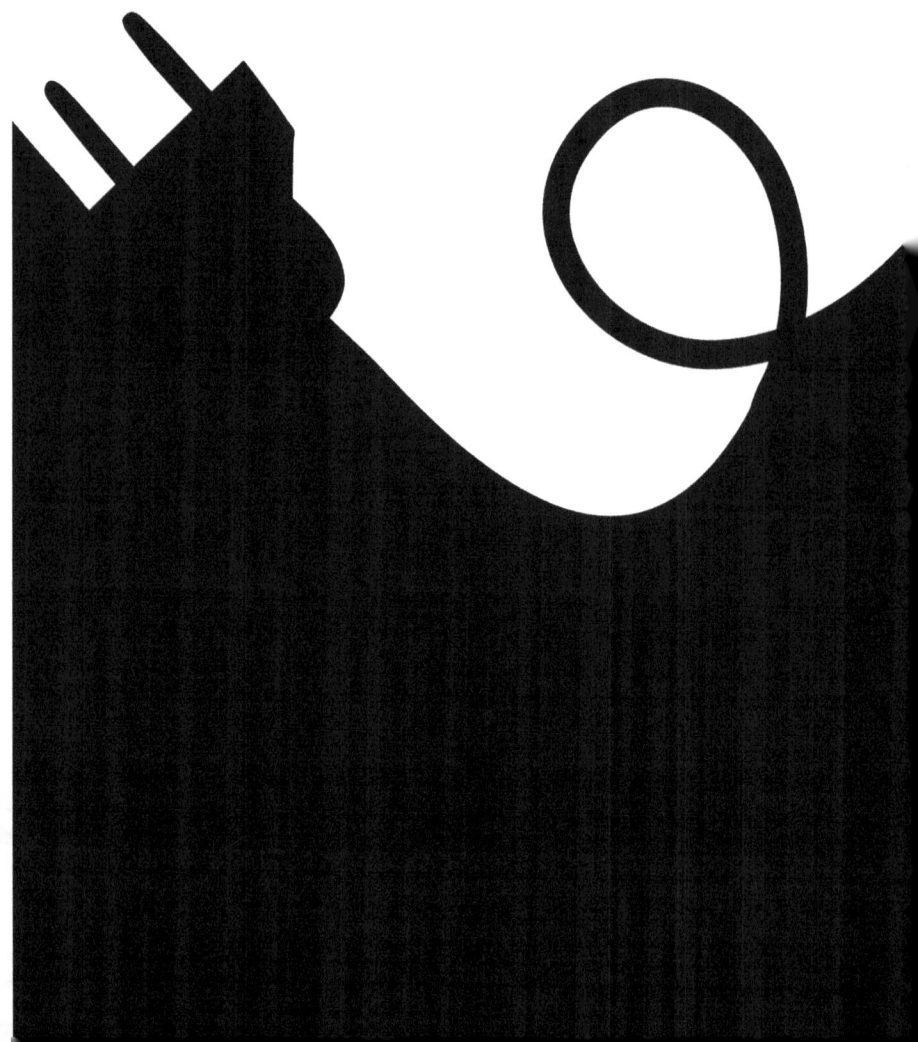

DAILY GRATITUDE

What are three things you are grateful for today?

Who made a difference in your life today?

What was the best part of your day?

Describe your overall mood today in 1-3 words.

Today's Date

_____

_____

_____

_____

_____

_____

_____

_____

_____

_____

_____

_____

MY DREAMS ARE
ATTAINABLE

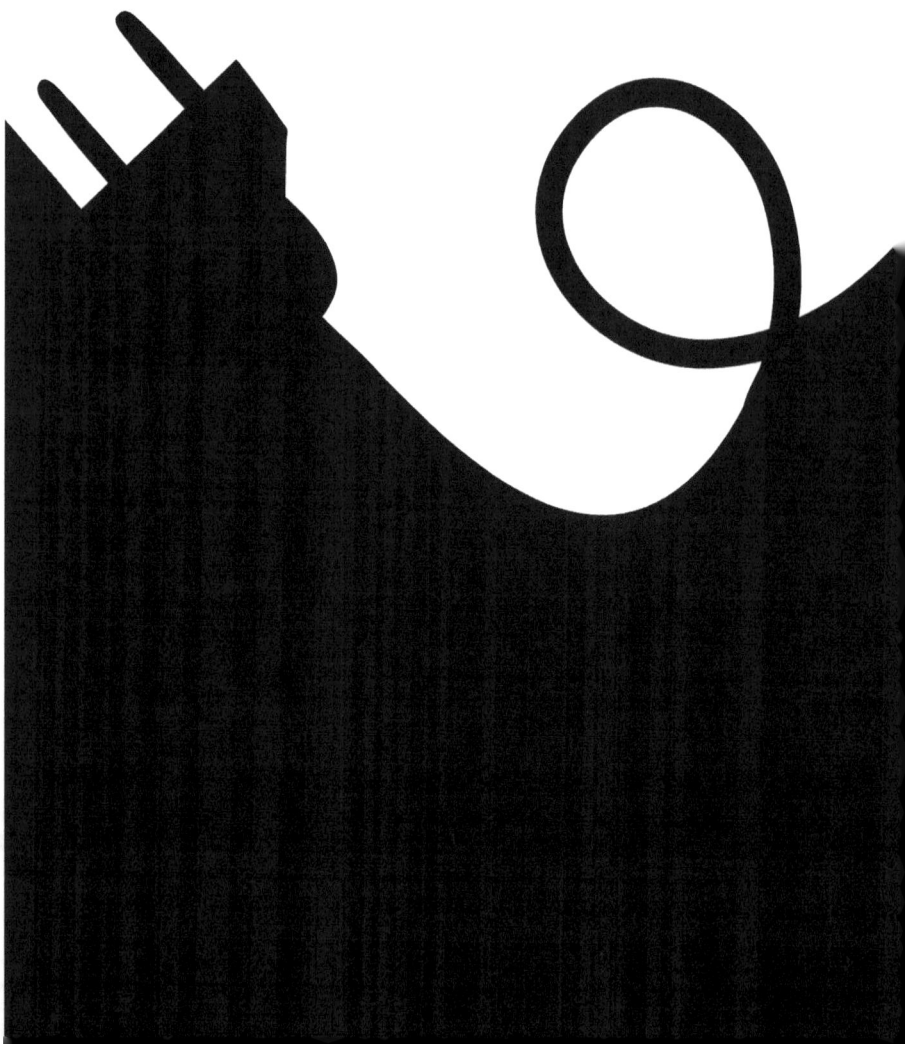

DAILY GRATITUDE

What are three things you are grateful for today?

Who made a difference in your life today?

What was the best part of your day?

Describe your overall mood today in 1-3 words.

Today's Date

IT'S OKAY TO
TAKE DEEP
BREATHS WHEN
I NEED TO

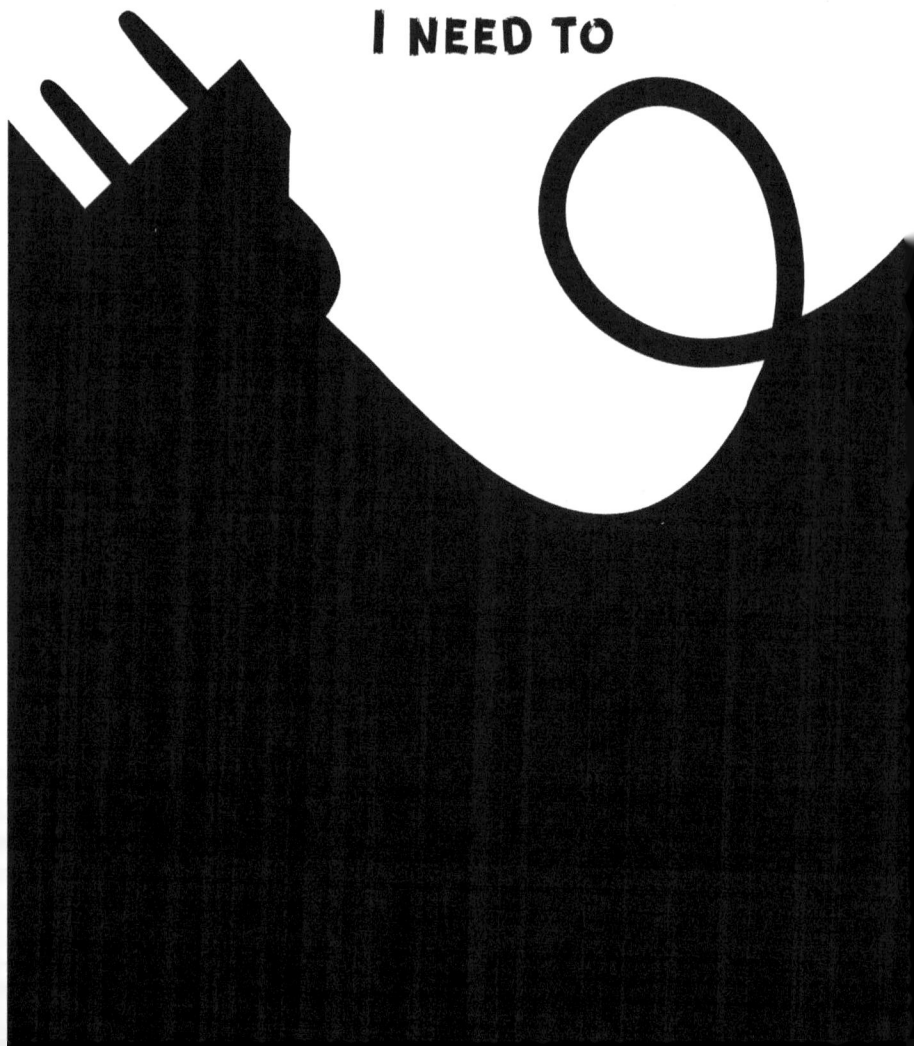

DAILY GRATITUDE

What are three things you are grateful for today?

Who made a difference in your life today?

What was the best part of your day?

Describe your overall mood today in 1-3 words.

Today's Date

_____

_____

_____

_____

_____

_____

_____

_____

_____

_____

_____

_____

_____

_____

_____

_____

_____

_____

_____

_____
_____
_____
_____
_____
_____
_____
_____
_____
_____
_____
_____
_____
_____

I MAKE A
DIFFERENCE

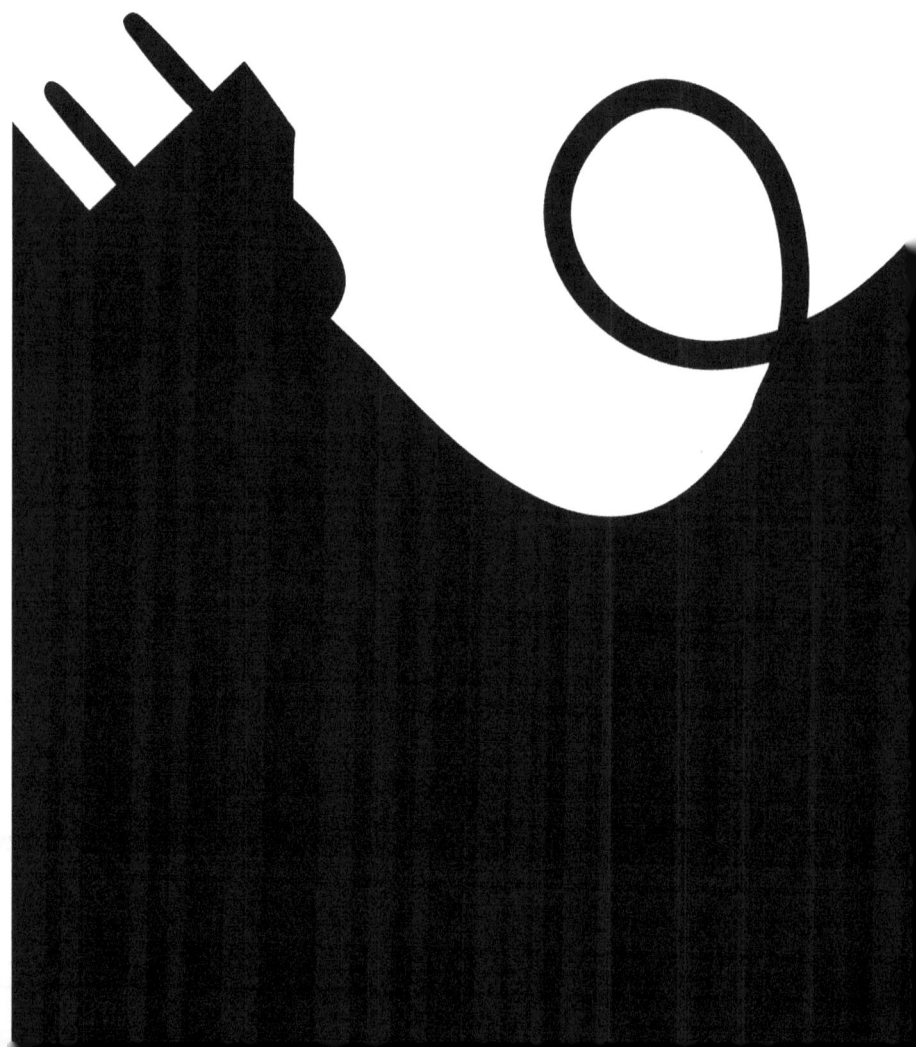

DAILY GRATITUDE

What are three things you are grateful for today?

Who made a difference in your life today?

What was the best part of your day?

Describe your overall mood today in 1-3 words.

Today's Date

IT'S GOOD TO SHARE
MY FEELINGS WITH
PEOPLE I CAN TRUST

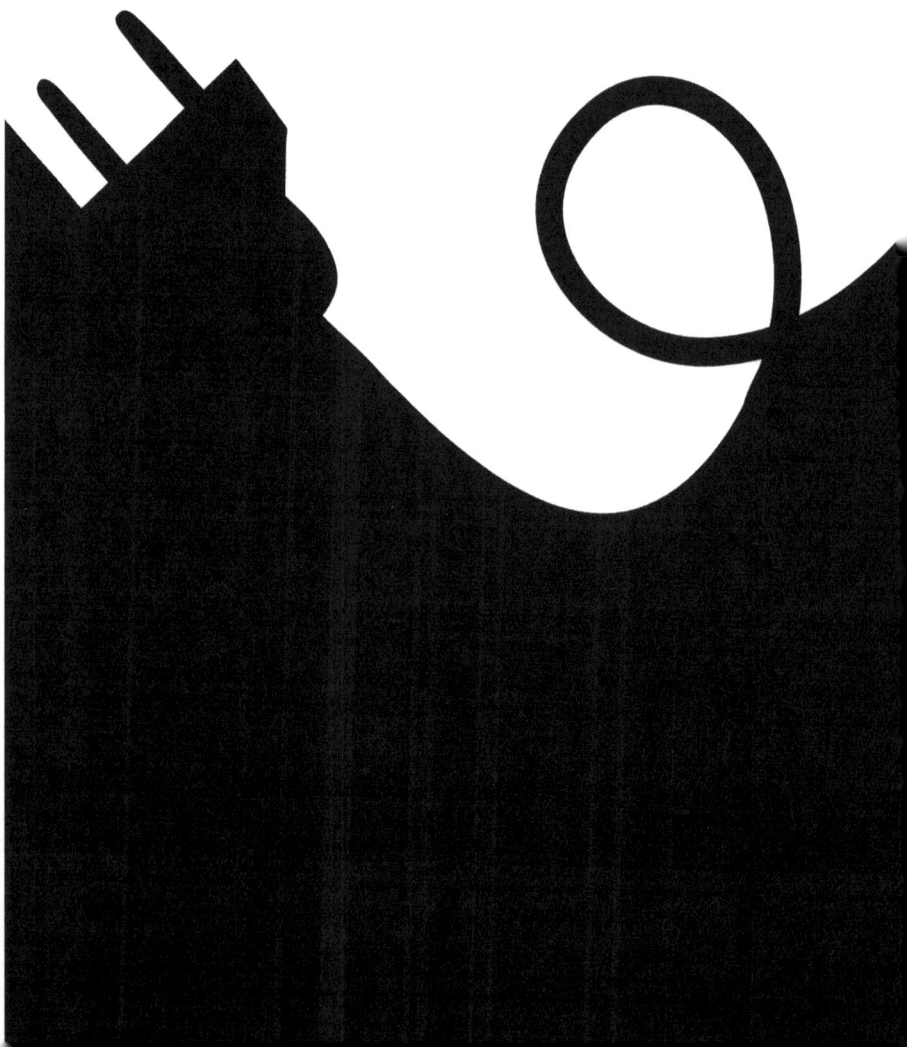

DAILY GRATITUDE

What are three things you are grateful for today?

Who made a difference in your life today?

What was the best part of your day?

Describe your overall mood today in 1-3 words.

Today's Date

TODAY, WRITE YOUR OWN AFFIRMATION IN
THE SPACE ABOVE.

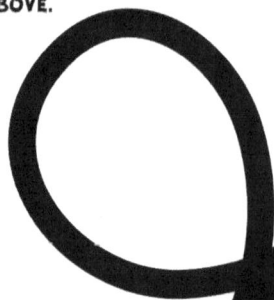

DAILY GRATITUDE

What are three things you are grateful for today?

Who made a difference in your life today?

What was the best part of your day?

Describe your overall mood today in 1-3 words.

Today's Date

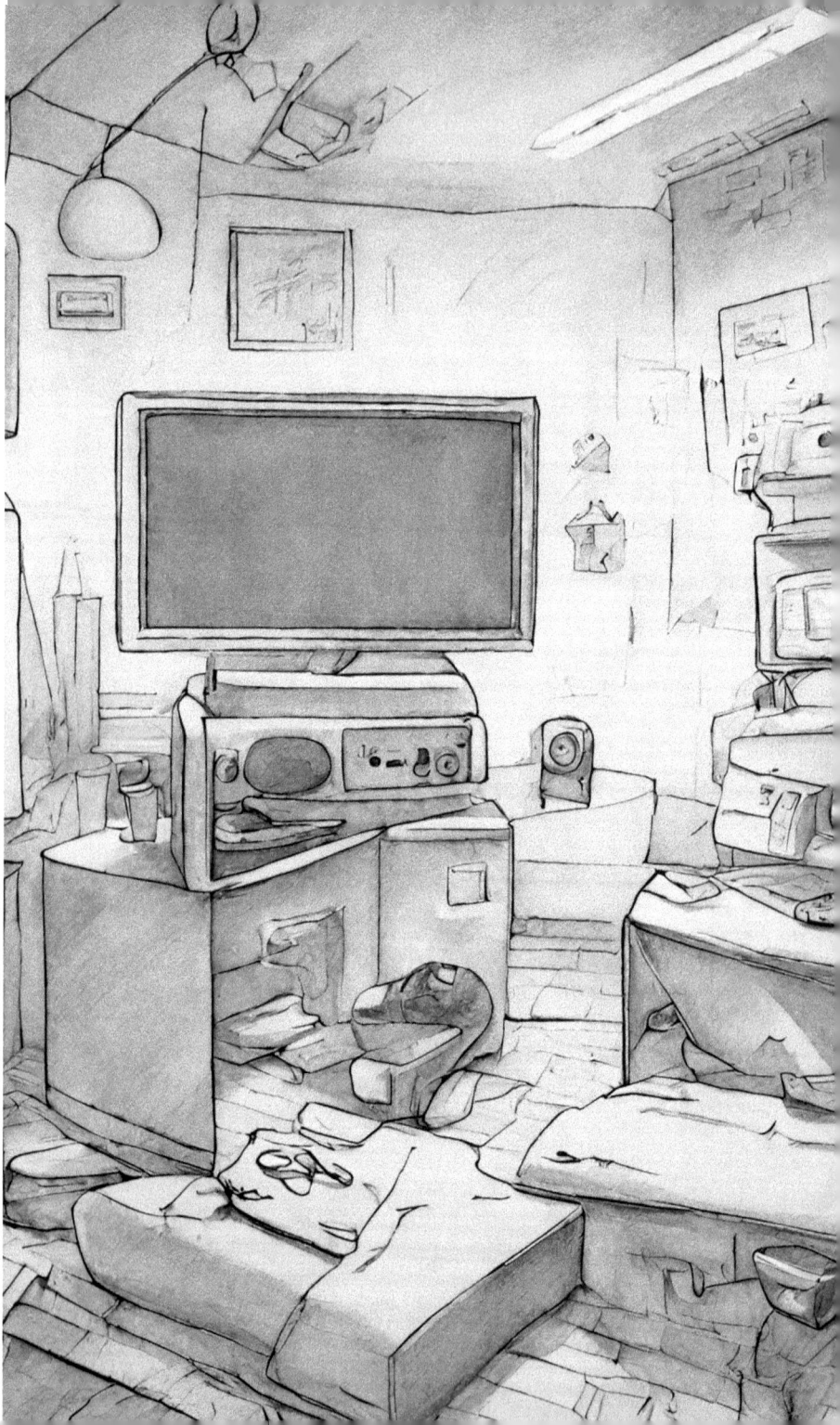

THINGS THAT MATTER

TO ME

LIST THREE PERSONAL OBJECTS THAT ARE MEANINGFUL.

1.
2.
3.

LIST THREE THING YOU HAVE THAT OTHERS DO NOT.

1.
2.
3.

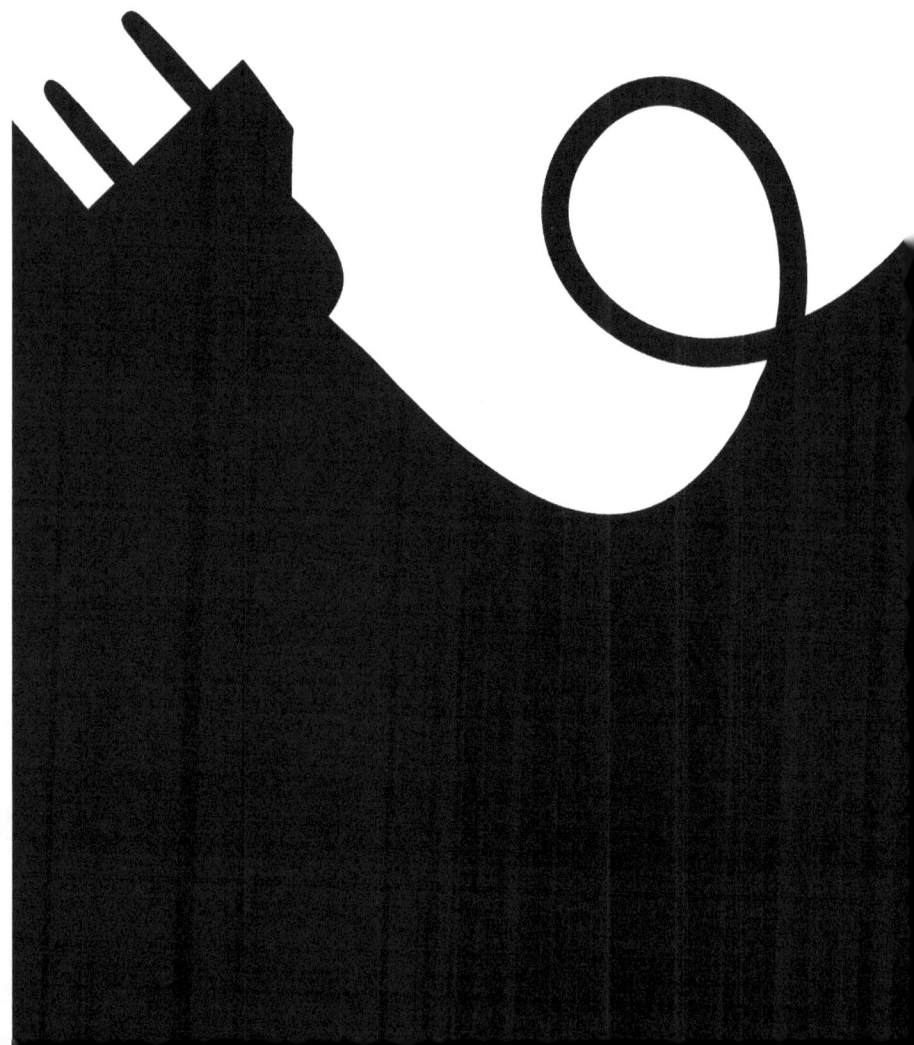

I STAND UP FOR
WHAT I BELIEVE
IN

DAILY GRATITUDE

What are three things you are grateful for today?

Who made a difference in your life today?

What was the best part of your day?

Describe your overall mood today in 1-3 words.

Today's Date

I AM A GOOD FRIEND, NOT A BULLY

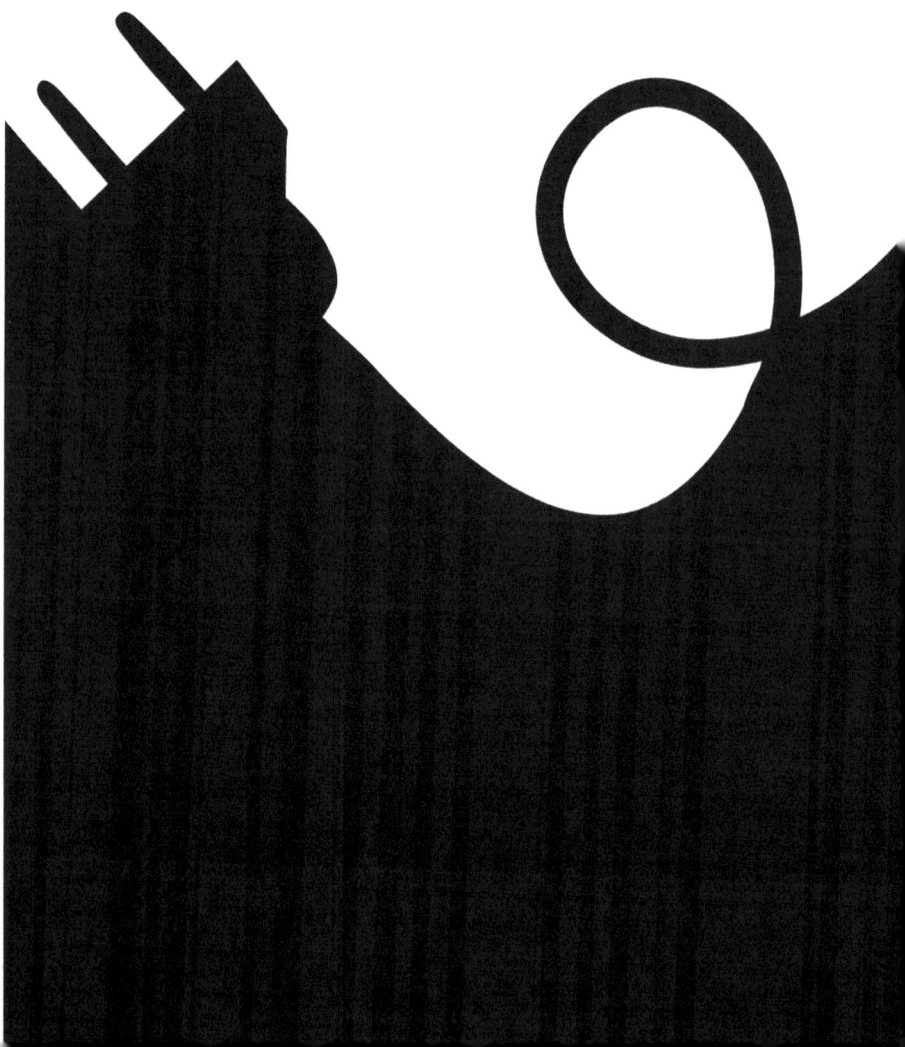

DAILY GRATITUDE

What are three things you are grateful for today?

Who made a difference in your life today?

What was the best part of your day?

Describe your overall mood today in 1-3 words.

Today's Date

THINGS A FRIEND WILL DO:

THINGS A FRIEND WILL SAY:

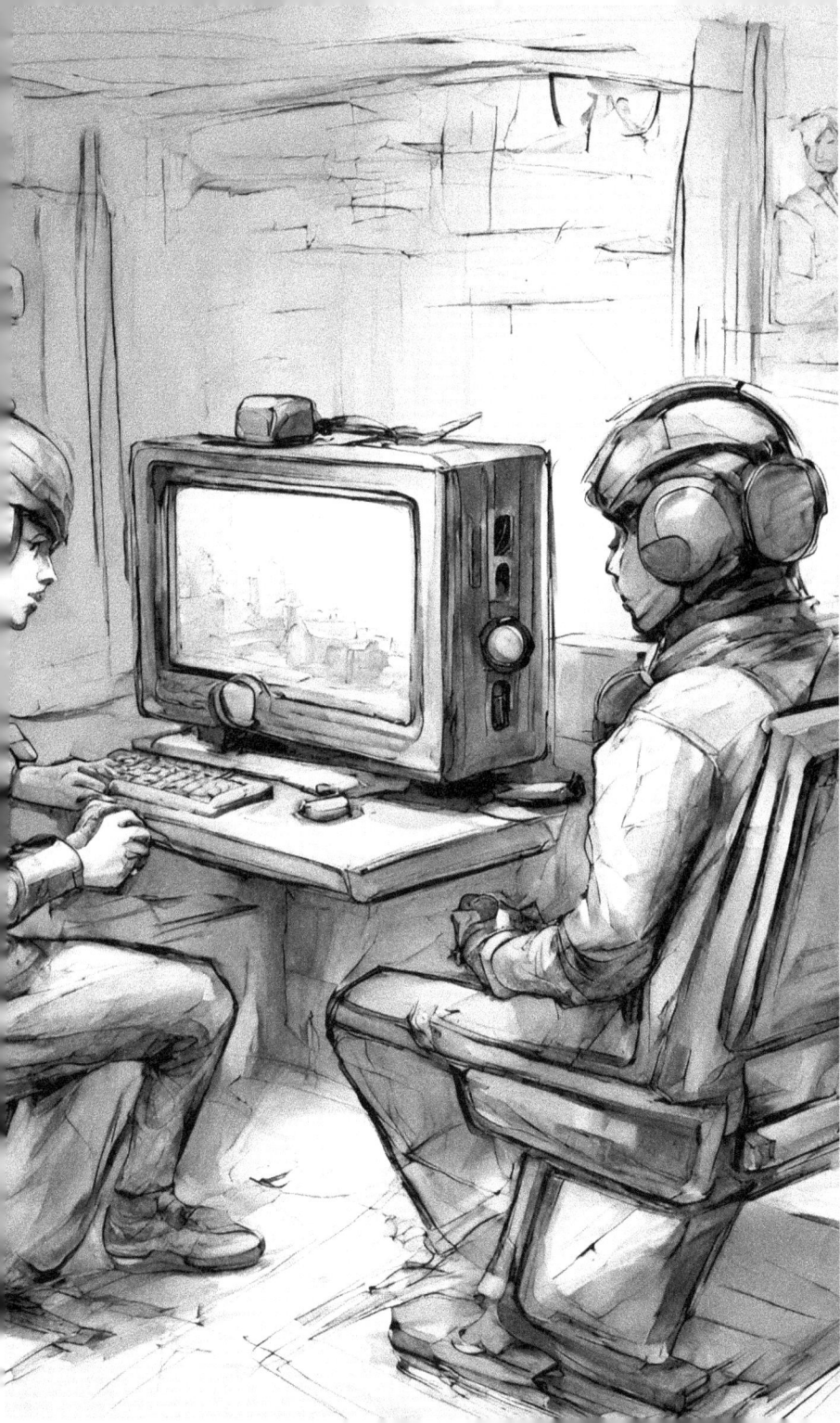

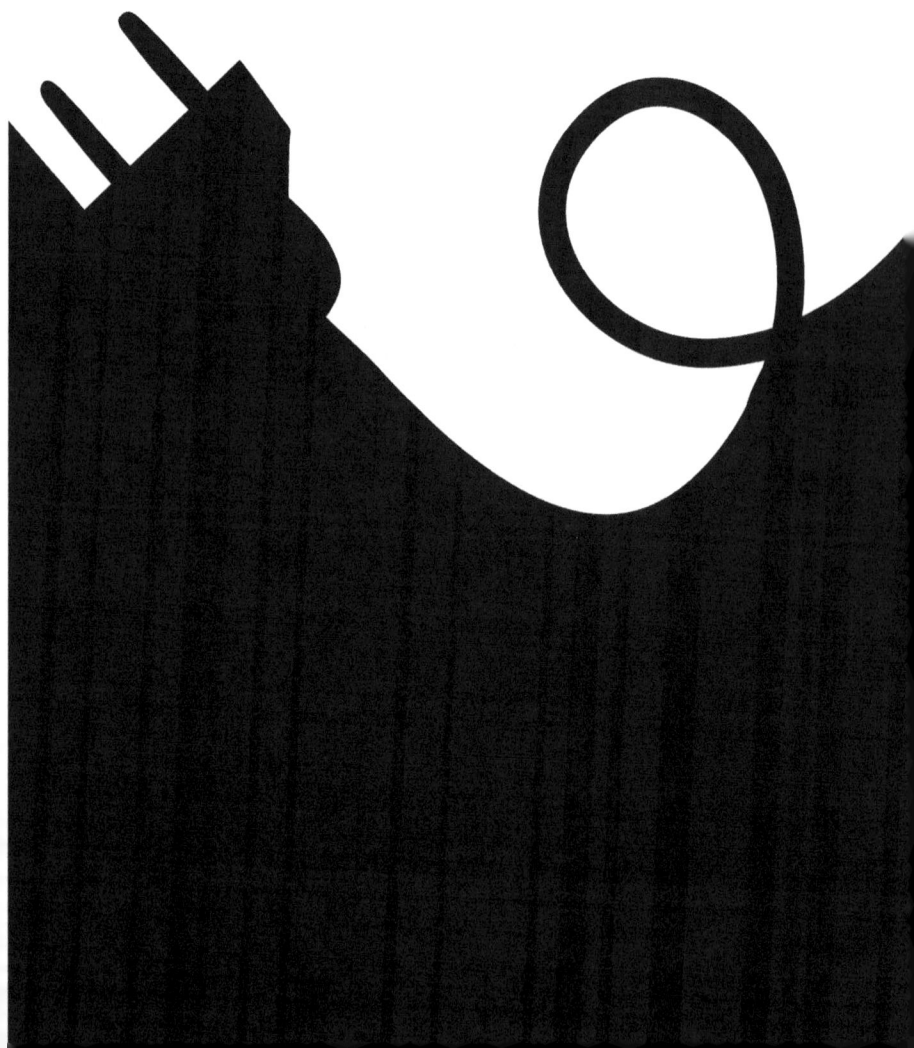

I AM KIND

DAILY GRATITUDE

What are three things you are grateful for today?

Who made a difference in your life today?

What was the best part of your day?

Describe your overall mood today in 1-3 words.

Today's Date

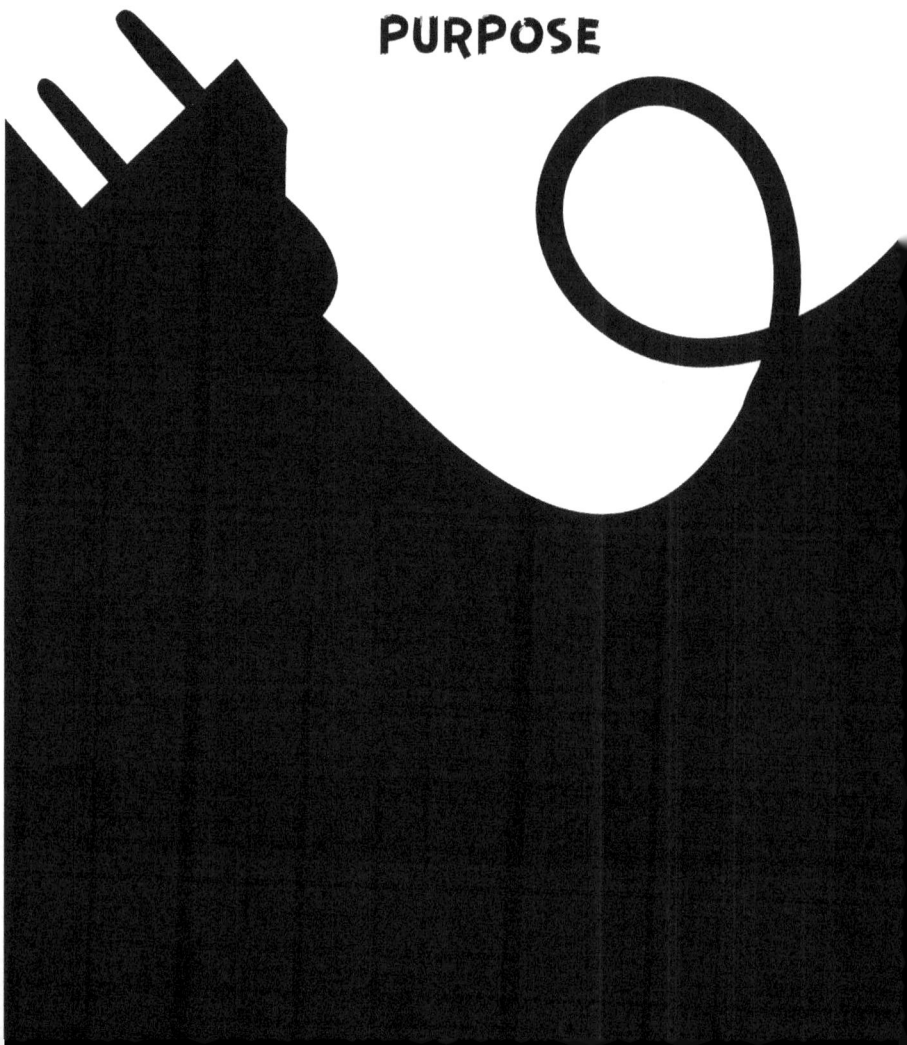

I WAS CREATED FOR A WONDERFUL PURPOSE

DAILY GRATITUDE

What are three things you are grateful for today?

Who made a difference in your life today?

What was the best part of your day?

Describe your overall mood today in 1-3 words.

Today's Date

_____

_____

_____

_____

_____

_____

_____

_____

_____

_____

_____

_____

_____

I CAN FACE MY FEARS

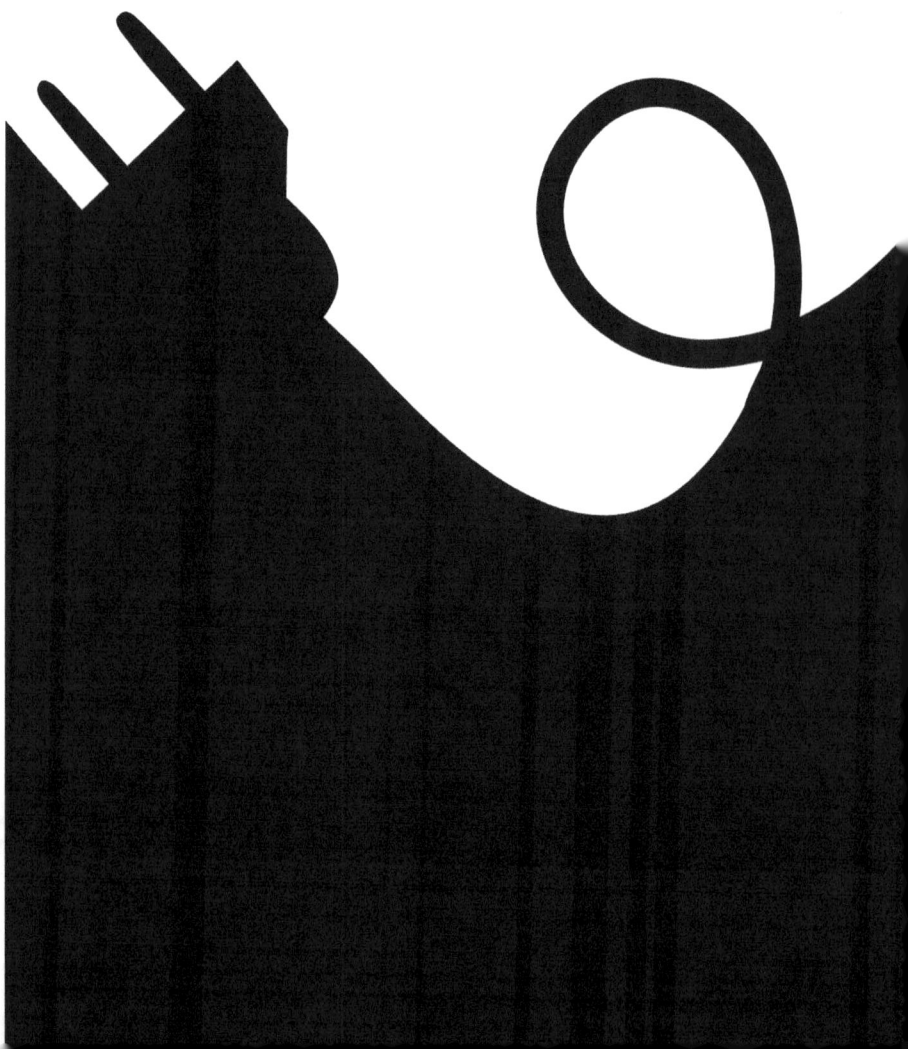

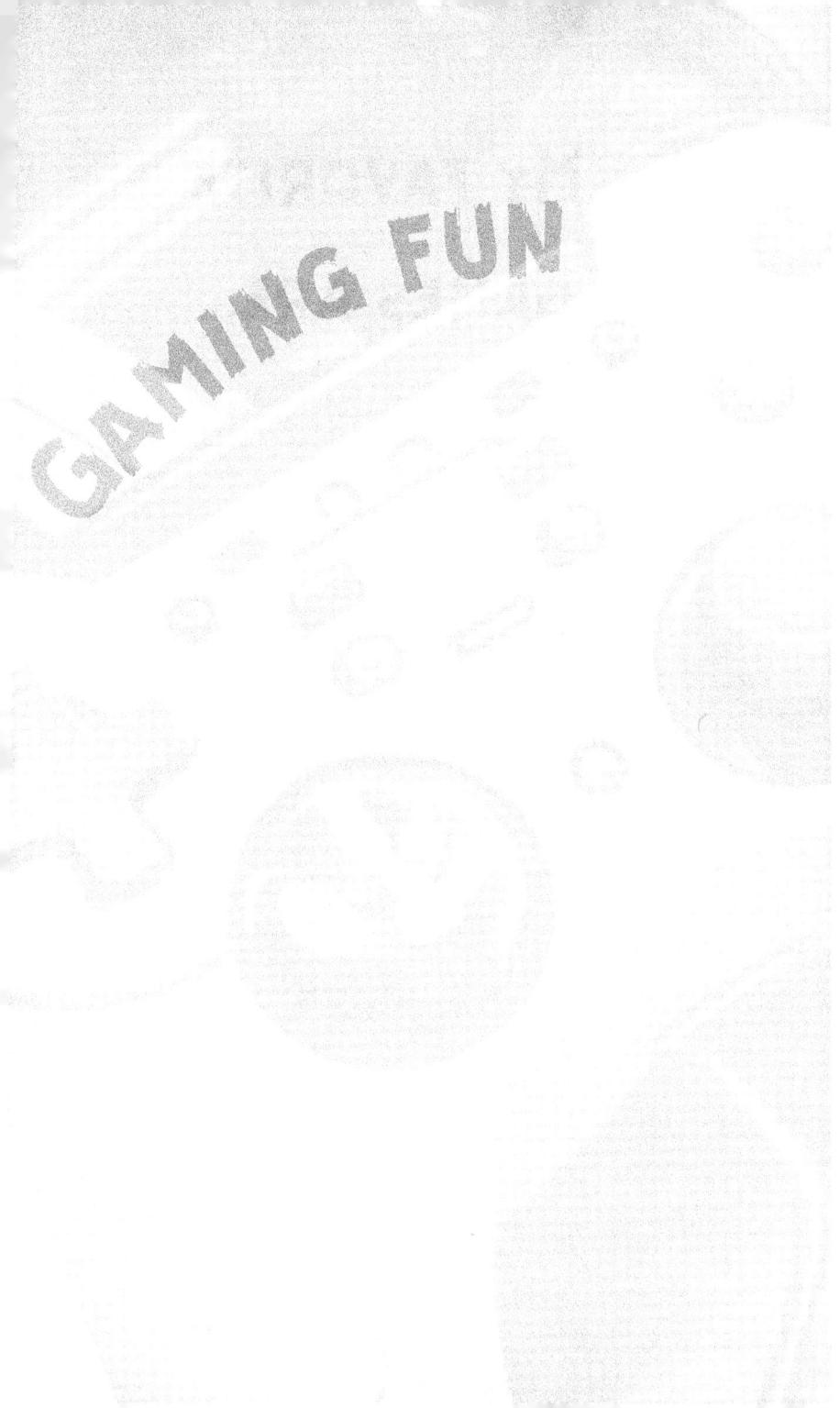

GAMING FUN

MY FAVORITE GAMES ARE...

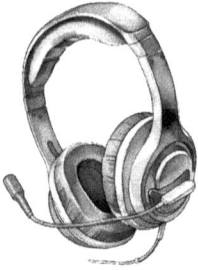

- ☐ ....
- ☐ ....
- ☐ ....
- ☐ ....
- ☐ ....
- ☐ ....
- ☐ ....
- ☐ ....
- ☐ ....
- ☐ ....

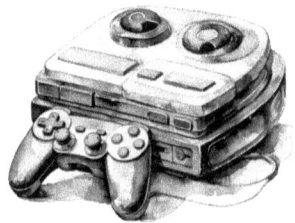

Video Game Review

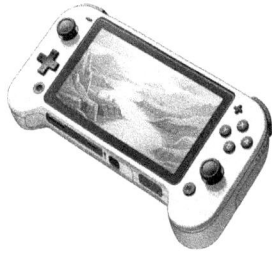

GAME

CREATOR

GRAPHICS

CHAIRS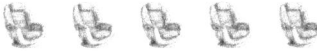

RECORD OF SCORE

BEST PART OF THE GAME:

Other Thoughts

Favorite Game Quotes

GAME

QUOTE

GAME

QUOTE

GAME

QUOTE

GAME

QUOTE

GAME

QUOTE

More Titles by Marya

SELF-HELP & GROWTH

Into the Water: Wading Through Grief
Out of the Water: a Baptism Devotional
Playing in the Dirt & Loving It
Gratitude is the Way
One Year Growth, (peacock-themed) Journal
Autism Love: Journal for Caregivers
Every Crown Has a Story: Tell Your Hair-Story
Be a Pink Dolphin

CHILDREN'S BOOKS

Time to Dance (2-9 years)
Small Big Gifts (1-6 years)

PRAYER JOURNALS

Prayer & Self-Care for Black Women
Prayer & Self-Care for Black Men
Prayer & Self-Care for Women
Prayer & Self-Care for Men

THEMED FULL-COLOR PERSONAL JOURNALS

Butterfly Bliss	Plant Love in Blue
Sunny Days.	Plant Lovers Journal
Magical Moments with Unicorns.	Time to Dream (unicorns)

THEMED BLACK & WHITE PERSONAL JOURNALS

That Black Cat	Crazy Plant Lady Journal
I Heart Dogs.	Book Club Journal
I Heart Horses	Reading Log Journal
Black Girl Magic: Mermaids	Prompts for Creative Writers

VISIT: TIME2DANCE.ORG

@author.maryapatricesherron

www.ingramcontent.com/pod-product-compliance
Lightning Source LLC
Chambersburg PA
CBHW070120030426
42335CB00016B/2214